Free Radicals Effect on Cytostatica, Vitamins, Hormones and Phytocompounds with Respect to Cancer: An Introduction to Molecular Radiation Biology

Free Radicals Effect on Cytostatica, Vitamins, Hormones and Phytocompounds with Respect to Cancer: An Introduction to Molecular Radiation Biology

Nikola Getoff

For permission to use material from this book please contact us:
Telephone 631-231-7269; Fax 631-231-8175
Web Site: http://www.novapublishers.com

Library of Congress Cataloging-in-Publication Data

etoff, Nikola, 1922-
Free radicals effect on cytostatica, vitamins, hormones and phytocompounds with respect to cancer / Nikola Getoff (author). p. ; cm.
Includes bibliographical references and index.
ISBN 978-1-60456-291-0 (hardcover)
1. Antineoplastic agents. 2. Cancer--Molecular aspects. 3. Free radicals (Chemistry) 4. Vitamins. 5. Antioxidants. I. Title.
[DNLM: 1. Antineoplastic Agents--pharmacology. 2. Free Radicals--metabolism. 3. Antioxidants--pharmacology. 4. Pulse Radiolysis--methods. 5. Vitamins--pharmacology. QV 269 G394f 2008]
RC271.C5G48 2008
616.99'4061--dc22 *2008023108*

Published by Nova Science Publishers, Inc. ≃ New York

Contents

Preface

The present book is derived from lectures on molecular radiation biology given for years, to students at the University of Vienna, in addition to intense research work performed in the field. The basis for this modern and very promising scientific field is the fact, that free radicals generated in human organism, can also be produced by action of ionizing radiation in isolated aqueous systems. Hence, the knowledge of the fundamental radiation chemistry of biological substances, combined with those of certain areas of biology, medicine and related domains, represent the frame of this young discipline. The molecular radiation biology has benefited very much from a number of experimental methods, which were successfully adopted from other disciplines. Its research area embraces a good deal of other medicine problems, particularly the combat of cancer in addition to the elucidation of biological reaction mechanisms induced by free radicals.

The book represents an attempt to demonstrate the advantage of new combined pathways of approach, showing particularly the importance of knowledge about the biological effect and consequences of free radicals action in organism. It is hoped, that it will contribute and initiate more research work in this field.

It is for me a pleasant duty to express my great appreciation to my co-workers, Dr. Ruth Maria Quint for her extremely valuable help recording the manuscript of the book on computer and Mr. Johannes Hartmann assisting me in the literature search. Last but not least, I like to thank my family for the forbearance and understanding during the time of book writing.

The author
Vienna, February 2008

Chapter 1

Introduction

The aim of this book is to present the actual knowledge and experiences gained in the interface field of molecular radiation biology and a special part of the oncology, embracing the effect of vitamins, cytostatica, hormones and phytocompounds. The subject is based on the fact, that the oxidizing (e.g. OH, $O_2^{\bullet-}$ etc.) and reducing free radicals (e_{aq}^-, H etc.), generated in human organism, by enzymatic, redox and many other processes, can be also produced and studied by deposition of radiation energy in appropriate aqueous systems. In such case the specific biological action of each desired kind of radicals on a given substrate can be investigated out of the organism. This offers the possibility to study the reaction mechanisms of the individual free radicals, resulting from water radiolysis, with above mentioned compounds. In addition, if the occasion should arise, also the synergistic effects between the involved substrates can be examined.

Beyond that by combination of the results obtained by pulse radiolysis technique (spectroscopic and kinetic characterization of free radicals) with those gained by experiments in vitro and chemical analysis of final products originating from the substrates, one can get a deeper insight and better understanding of the fast and complicated biological processes. Therefore, the so obtained results may contribute to a more successful therapy of cancer and other illnesses.

As an introduction to the subject matter some basic knowledge of radion chemistry / radiation biology, such as water radiolysis (human organism consists of about 70% water), photochemical and biological formation of "solvated electrons" (e_{aq}^-), ozone-species and free radicals data determined by pulse radiolysis is presented. The last method is frequently implemented for more precise studies of transients and is playing a significant role in radiation biology. ESR-method is not included here, although it is in some cases useful.

The results concerning the synergistic effect of vitamins with cytostatica, mitomycin C (MMC) and procarbacine (PC) are reported as examples for illustration of the subject matter. Hence, the transients of these drugs studied by pulse radiolysis are reviewed. Subsequently, the species resulting from the antioxidant vitamins (C,E and β-carotene), as well as their combined protection action of the cell membrane are discussed. The synergistic effect of these three vitamins on the cytostatica efficiency is demonstrated by experiments in vitro. The peculiar antitumor as well as synergistic behaviour of the vitamins of the B-series (B1 to B6) is individually discussed. Special attention is, however, given to vitamin B11 (folic acid), where very fast intramolecular electron transfer processes within the life-time of its transients are observed.These facts are reflecting the many-sided action of the vitamin transients. The role of some other vitamins (A,D etc.) in respect to cancer were also briefly discussed. In addition data concerning the individual biological behaviour of some sexual hormones, particularly 17β-estradiol in relation to breast cancer, as well as the multi-action of phytocompounds (resveratrol, genistein, inositol) and their synergistic effect on cytostatica are reported.

Ultimately, two rather important factors as possible initiators for carcinogenesis, namely the effect of environmental influences and nutrition are also mentioned.

For the sake of completeness to the text of the book also tables and figures of useful physical data, absorption spectra and spectroscopic characteristics of the primary products of water radiolysis etc. are given as an appendix.

Chapter 2

Free Radicals

Generally, free radicals and radical ions can be generated by deposition of energy in a system, which is enough to cause splitting of a chemical bond or to transfer an electron. In human organism such processes can be induced by biological systems (enzymes, hormones, redox-reactions etc.), where most frequently trace element-ions (Fe^{2+}, Zn^{2+}, Mg^{2+}, Co^{2+}, Mn^{2+} etc.) act as catalysts and render such reactions at lower energy. On the other hand even under normal conditions oxygen is in electronically excited triplet state, which makes it possible to initiate and/or contribute to such processes. In addition to this, short lived species can be also formed under the influence of solar energy, uv-light, microwave radiation, laser and ionizing radiation (high energy electrons, gamma and X-ray etc.). In the present essay ionizing radiation in respect to radiation therapy of cancer will be mostly concerned. The discussed processes, however, are also valid for the chemotherapy likewise, since as mentioned above, the same free radicals initiating the processes under irradiation are also generated biologically in the human organism.

2.1. Water Radiolysis

The human organism consists of about 70% water. Under the influence of ionizing radiation the energy is deposited in about 10^{-15} s in the media, where the water molecules become either electronically excited (H_2O^*) or ionized ($H_2O^{\bullet+}$, e^-). The H_2O^* molecules can decompose to H and OH radicals or deactivate, following photophysical processes (luminescence and radiationless deactivation). Simultaneously, each radical cation, $H_2O^{\bullet+}$, can react with a neutral water molecule, resulting into OH radical and hydronium ion ($H_3O^+ = H_{aq}^+$). By interaction with the media the primary produced electrons lose very rapidly their energy upto ≤ 10 eV (forming further ecxited and ionizied water molecules) and become "thermalyzed electrons" (e_{th}^-). Based on their polar nature, water molecules rearrange their dipoles around each e_{th}^- within about $2x10^{-12}$ s, forming "solvated electrons" (e_{aq}^-). The solvated electrons (e_{aq}^-) represent the basic form of the reducing species and opposite, the H atoms are their acid form. The produced OH, H and e_{aq}^- can react very fast with each other resulting into the "molecular products", H_2, H_2O_2 and OH_{aq}^-. Therefore, as a result of the interaction of the ionizing radiation with water primary reducing (H, e_{aq}^-) and oxidizing (OH) free radicals and molecular products are formed (see e.g. /1-3/). The primary products of water radiolysis react rather fast with each other and with the molecular products (H_2 and H_2O_2), formed along the electron spur. Hence, at low substrate concentration these reactions can successfully compete with the solute.

The water radiolysis and the yields (G-values) of the primary radiolytic products as well as some transformation reactions of H and e_{aq}^- species are presented in Table 2.1. for completeness of the subject matter.

Some further data concerning the individual absorption spectra of the primary products, the reactions between them and the pH-dependence of their yields are presented in the appendix.

In the frame of pulse radiolysis studies (see later) and especially in experiments in vitro it is frequently desirable to investigate the individual biological action of a primary radical (OH, e_{aq}^- or H) with a given substrate. Hence, the reducing species, H and e_{aq}^-, can be converted into oxidizing ones ($HO_2^{\bullet}$ and $O_2^{\bullet -}$) in the presence of air. By saturating the aqueous media with N_2O (~ 10^{-2} mol/L at room temperature) the strong reducing e_{aq}^- are transformed into the strongly oxidizing OH radicals. In aqueous solution containing sufficient concentration of H_2 (at high pressure) the OH species are converted into H atoms (see Table 2.1. and appendix).

In aqueous solutions containing a calculated amount of formate or isopropanol, both OH and H are scavenged. The produced transients can thereafter transfer electrons to a substrate (RH), assuming that it has an appropriate rate constant (k) of the process, e.g.:

$$HCOO^- + OH \rightarrow {}^{\bullet}COO^- + H_2O \; (k = 2.7x10^9 \; L.mol^{-1}.s^{-1}) \quad (2.1)$$

$$HCOO^- + H \rightarrow {}^{\bullet}COO^- + H_2 \; (k = 2.5x10^7 \; L.mol^{-1}.s^{-1}) \quad (2.2)$$

$${}^{\bullet}COO^- + RH \rightarrow RH^{\bullet -} + CO_2 \quad (2.3)$$

$$(CH_3)_2CHOH + OH \rightarrow (CH_3)_2CHO^{\bullet} + H_2O \qquad (k = 2x10^9 \; L.mol^{-1}.s^{-1}) \quad (2.4)$$

$$(CH_3)_2CHOH + H \rightarrow (CH_3)_2CHO^{\bullet} + H_2 \; (k = 7{,}4x10^7 \; L.mol^{-1}.s^{-1}) \quad (2.5)$$

$$(CH_3)_2CHO^{\bullet} + RH \rightarrow RH^{\bullet -} + CH_3COCH_3 + H^+ \quad (2.6)$$

Naturally, these reactions are applicable under the supposition, that the resulting final products (CO_2 and acetone) are not essentially involved in the corresponding process. This can be, however, examined by chemical analysis of the resulting products. The probability of the involved competition reactions can be calculated by knowing the corresponding rate constants (k) and the concentrations of the implemented substrates. An excellent compilation of the rate constants for reactions of e_{aq}^-, H and $OH/O^{\bullet -}$ radicals with a large number of inorganic and organic compounds in aqueous solution is published by Buxton et al. /4/.

Table 2.1. Water radiolysis

Primary reactions:

$$H_2O \rightsquigarrow H_2O^* \rightarrow H + OH$$
$$\qquad\qquad\quad \rightarrow H_2O^+ + e^-;$$
$$e^- \rightarrow e_{th}^- + n\,H_2O \rightarrow e_{aq}^-$$

$$H_2O^+ + H_2O \rightarrow H_3O^+ + OH$$

Gross reaction of water radiolysis (the G-values*) at pH 7 are given in brackets):

$$H_2O \rightsquigarrow e_{aq}^-,\ H,\ OH,\ H_2,\ H_2O_2,\ H_{aq}^+,\ OH_{aq}^-$$

at pH = 6 to 8.5; G = (2.7) (0.6) (2.8) (0.45) (0.7) (3.2) (0.5)

$OH_{aq}^- + H_{aq}^+ \rightarrow H_2O$ $(k = 1.4 \times 10^{11}\ L.mol^{-1}\ s^{-1})$

$e_{aq}^- + H_{aq}^+ \rightarrow H + H_2O$ $(k = 2.3 \times 10^{10}\ L.mol^{-1}\ s^{-1})$

$H + OH_{aq}^- \rightarrow e_{aq}^-$ $(k = 2.2 \times 10^{7}\ L.mol^{-1}\ s^{-1})$

$OH \rightleftharpoons H_{aq}^+ + O_{aq}^{\bullet -}$ $(pK = 11.9)$

$H_2O_2 \rightleftharpoons H_{aq}^+ + HO_{2,aq}^-$ $(pK = 11.65)$

In the presence of oxygen:

$H + O_2 \rightarrow HO_2^{\bullet}$ $(k = 2 \times 10^{10}\ L.mol^{-1}\ s^{-1})$

$e_{aq}^- + O_2 \rightarrow O_2^{\bullet -}$ $(k = 1.9 \times 10^{10}\ L.mol^{-1}\ s^{-1})$

$HO_2^{\bullet} \rightleftharpoons H^+ + O_2^{\bullet -}$ $(pK = 4.8)$

In the presence of N_2O:

$e_{aq}^- + N_2O \rightarrow OH + OH^- + N_2$ $(k = 0.91 \times 10^{10}\ L.mol^{-1}\ s^{-1})$

In the presence of H_2:

$OH + H_2 \rightarrow H_2O + H$ $(k = 3.5 \times 10^{7}\ L.mol^{-1}\ s^{-1})$

MEDIUM (pH = 6.4 – 8.6)

Airfree	Air	N_2O
46% OH 44% e^-_{aq} 10% H	46% OH 54% $O_2^{\bullet -}$	90% OH 10% H

*) G-value = number of changed molecules per 100 eV (1.60×10^{-17} J) absorbed energy. For conversion into SI-units: multiply the G-value by 0.10364 to obtain G(x) in μmol.J^{-1}.

1 Gy (Gray) = 100 rad = 6.24×10^{15} eV.g^{-1}.
1 Gy generate 6.344×10^{-7} mol.L^{-1} (e_{aq}^- + H + OH).

2.2. Water Photolysis

Water absorbs light in vacuum-uv-range ($\lambda \leq 200$ nm) /5/. As a suitable source for VUV-light, low pressure Hg-lamps are used, which are emitting simultaneously at $\lambda = 184$ nm (10%) and 253.7 nm (100%) (see e.g. /6/). For the production of vacuum-UV-light at 147 nm (8.4 eV/hν) and at 123.6 nm (10.4 eV/hν) special constructed electrodeless VUV-lamps, filled wilth 1 mm pressure of Xenon or Krypton, respectively are available (Figure 2.2.1.) They are driven by a microwave-generator /7/.

The water can be decomposed by VUV-light leading to the same primary products (OH, H, e_{aq}^-) as by ionizing radiation. However, the yields are different, depending on the applied energy of the VUV-light. The excited water molecules (H_2O^*) can decompose to H and OH radicals or/and can lead to the formation of "super excited" water molecules (H_2O^{**}). The last ones can lead to formation of e_{aq}^-, since the absorbed energy exceeds the ionization potential of water (12.6 eV) /8/ and refs. therein/.

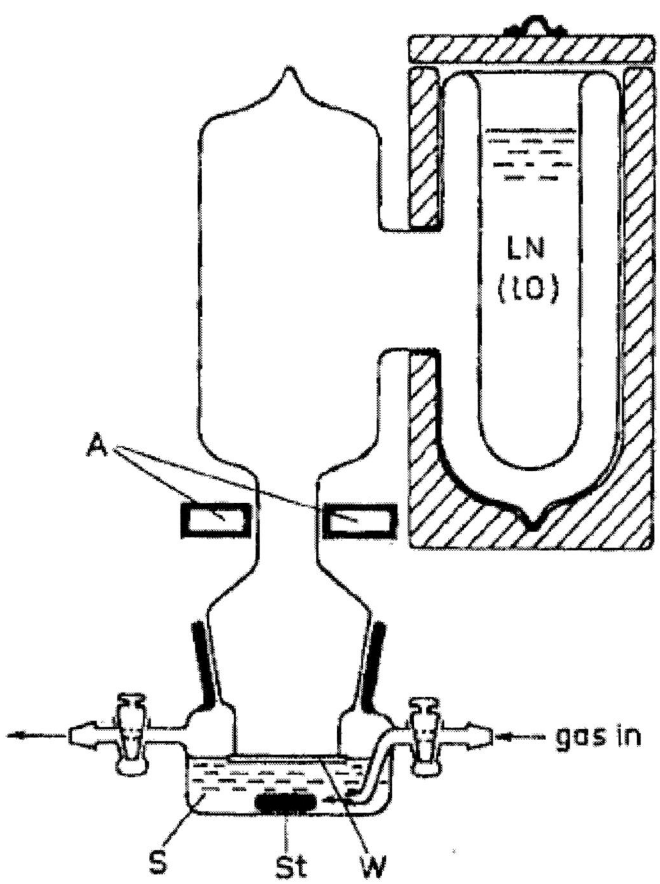

Figure 2.2.1. VUV-lamp for irradiation of liquids, equipped with MgF_2-window, which is transparent for VUV-light /7/, where: S .. solution, St .... stirrer, W .... window from MgF_2, LN ... liquid nitrogen, LO ... liquid oxygen.

$$H_2O \rightsquigarrow H_2O^* \rightarrow H + O \qquad (2.2.1)$$

$$H_2O^* + H_2O^* \rightarrow H_2O + H_2O^{**} \qquad (2.2.2)$$

$$H_2O^{**} \rightarrow H_2O + e_{aq}^- \qquad (2.2.3)$$

The quantum yields (Q) of the primary products at various wavelengths are given in Table 2.2.1.

Table 2.2.1. Quantum yields of photolytic primary products obtained at various VUV wavelengths as well as calculated G_{ph}-values related to 100 eV absorbed VUV-light

VUV	Energy	Q-yields			G_{ph}-yields		
λ [nm]	eV/hν	H	OH	e_{aq}^-	H	OH	e_{aq}^-
184.9	6.7	0.33	0.33	0.03	4.9	4.9	0.45
147	8.4	0.7	0.7	0.07	8.3	8.3	0.83
123.6	10.4	1.0	1.0	0.10	9.6	9.6	0.96

In order to compare the yields of the photolytic primary product, with those obtained by water radiolysis (Table 2.1.), the quantum yields given in Table 2.2.1 are calculated on the basis for 100 eV absorbed VUV-energy. The obtained "photochemical G-values" (G_{ph}) are also shown in Table 2.2.1. Obviously the G_{ph}-values of H and OH radicals are much higher than the corresponding values observed by water radiolysis , but the $G_{ph}(e_{aq}^-)$ are essential lower. This fact is related to the nature of both types of radiation.

The VUV-light emitted by the sun is absorbed in the atmosphere. The shortest wavelength reaching the earth surface amounts to λ = 315 nm (3.9 eV/hν).

2.3. Photochemical and Biological Formation of Solvated Electrons (E_{aq}^-)

It has been established, that "solvated electrons" (e_{aq}^-) can be also produced in aqueous solutions from electronically excited organic molecules at energies far below the ionization potential of the given compound. This fact is not only of chemical interest, but also biochemical, biological and even of medical importance (e.g. phototherapy of skin cancer etc.). In the frame of numerous photophysical investigations of organic substances it was found, that the yield of e_{aq}^- ejected from an organic molecule strongly depends on several factors, such as: electronic structure of the molecule, pH of the aqueous solution, temperature and especially on its substituents such as: -OH, $-O^-$, $-OCH_3$, $-OPO_3H_2$, $-OPO_3H^-$, $-COO^-$, -NH_2, $-NHCH_3$, $-N(CH_3)_2$, -SH etc.. These findings have been already discussed in a review article (/9/ and refs. therein).

Some experimental data in this respect may illustrate the relation between fluorescence and e_{aq}^-. First, it was proven, that both processes originate from the singlet excited state by using aqueous phenolate solution (pH > 12) as an electron donor and Cs^+ ions as a heavy atom fluorescence quencher. From the Stern-Volmer relationship (Figure2.3.1.) is clearly demonstrated, that both processes, e_{aq}^- and fluorescence are simultaneously quenched (quenching constant, K_{sv}= 5.2 mol^{-1}). This proves, that the electrons are also ejected directly from the singlet state, but not from the triplet state as previously postulated.

As well known aqueous phenol has a strongly fluorescence, but phenolate (pH > 10) shows extremely weak fluorescence. Studying both processes, fluorescence and electron yields, Q_F and $Q(e_{aq}^-)$ for aqueous phenol/phenolate in the pH-range from 1 to 13.6 it was established that Q_F-yield of phenol rapidly drops above pH > 8 (pK = 9.75), but at the same time the $Q(e_{aq}^-)$ yield, like mirror-image, is increasing (see Figure 2.3.2.). This demonstrate that the absorbed energy in the π-electron structure of benzene ring in the case of phenol is mainly emitted as fluorescence, whereas the electron of the -O^- group in phenolate is ejected (formation of e_{aq}^-) on the expense of fluoresecence.

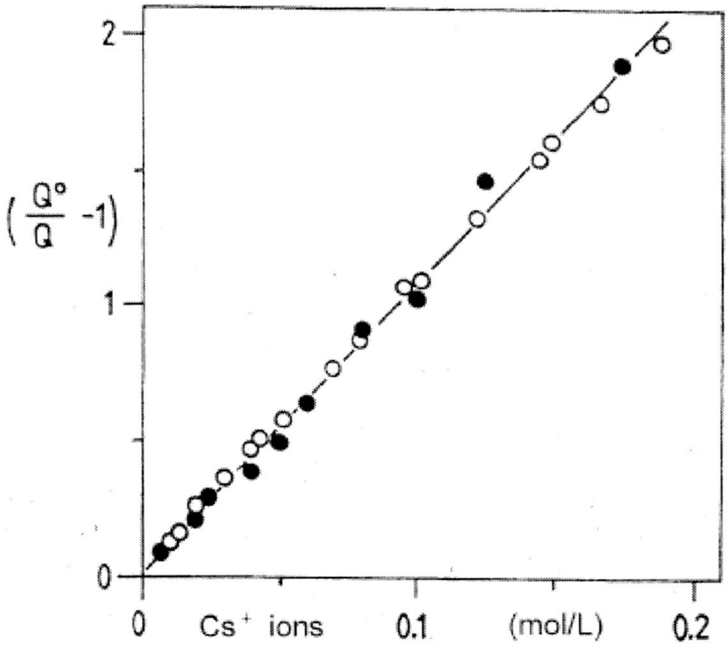

Figure 2.3.1. Stern-Volmer plot: quenching of fluorescence (o) and e_{aq}^- formation (●) of aqueous 10^{-2} mol/L phenol (pH ~ 7) by Cs^+-ions (OH-scavenger: 1 mol/L 2-propanol; e_{aq}^--scavenger: 2.8x10^{-2} mol/L N_2O; λ_{exc} = 254 nm). Q° is the quantum yield of fluorescence and e_{aq}^- without and Q in the presence of Cs^+-ions. (Reprint from Radiat.Phys.Chem.**34**, 711-719, 1989, by N.Getoff: A review of the relationship between $Q(e_{aq}^-)$ and Q_F of excited compounds in aqueous solution, with permission from Elsevier).

The effect of temperature on Q_F and $Q(e_{aq}^-)$ is illustrated in Figure 2.3.3. taking aqueous phenylphosphate as a model substrate. Here, again the energy of the UV-light (λ=254 nm) is absorbed practically by the benzene ring and the phosphate group is acting as electron donor. With increasing the temperature of the solution above 30°C the Q_F-value rapidly decreases,

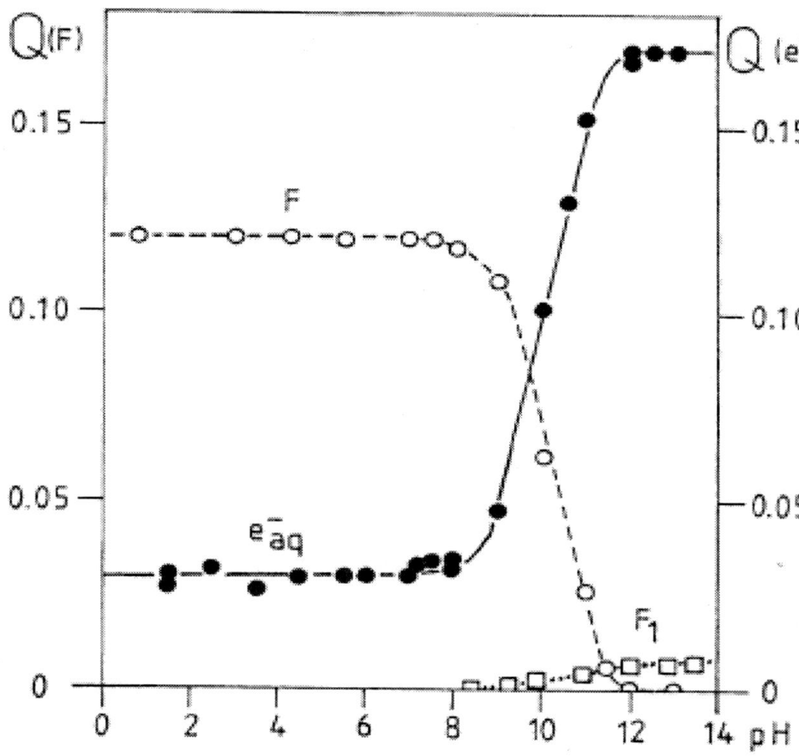

Figure 2.3.2. pH-Dependence of Q_F and $Q(e_{aq}^-)$ observed by UV-light (λ = 254 nm) of airfree aqueous 0.01 mol/L phenol or phenolate (pK = 9.75), 1 mol/L methanol and 0.028 mol/L N_2O at 30°C. (F) for phenol λ_{em} = 296 nm and (F_1) for phenolate λ_{em} = 336 nm. (Reprint from Radiat.Phys.Chem.**34**, 711-719, 1989, by N.Getoff: A review of the relationship between $Q(e_{aq}^-)$ and Q_F of excited compounds in aqueous solution, with permission from Elsevier).

but this of $Q(e_{aq}^-)$ is enhanced correspondently. This can be explained by the fact, that with the temperature increase the outer electron orbit of phosphate group is enlarged (weakening of the electron bonding energy). Simultaneously, the dipoles of the surrounding water molecules become oriented (in ~10^{-13} s) and interact with the electron of question, which finally become solvated (e_{aq}^-). This mechanism is graphically presented in Figure 2.3.4. taking aniline as a model /9/.

It should be also mentioned that various aqueous ions, like Cl_{aq}^-, $SO_{4,aq}^-$, Fe_{aq}^{2+} etc. can also lead to the formation of e_{aq}^- from their energetically excited state, e.g.:

$$Cl_{aq}^- + h\nu \rightarrow (Cl_{aq}^-)^* \rightarrow Cl^\bullet + e_{aq}^- \qquad (2.3.1.)$$

$$Cl^\bullet + nH_2O \rightarrow Cl_{aq}^- + H_{aq}^+ + OH \qquad (2.3.2.)$$

or:

$$Fe_{aq}^{2+} + h\nu \rightarrow (Fe_{aq}^{2+})^* \rightarrow Fe_{aq}^{3+} + e_{aq}^- \qquad (2.3.3.)$$

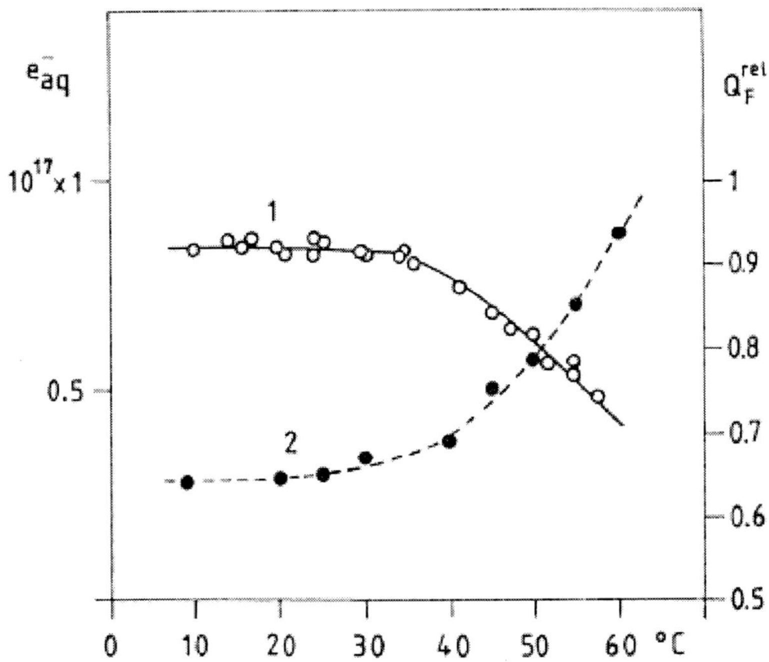

Figure 2.3.3. Temperature effect of fluorescence (Q_F^{rel}, curve 1) and e_{aq}^{-}-formation (number of e_{aq}^{-} per ml/min, curve 2) of aqueous 0.05 mol/L $C_6H_5OPO_3^{2-}$, 0.028 mol/L N_2O (scavenger of e_{aq}^{-}), UV-light λ_{exc}= 254 nm. (Reprint from Radiat.Phys.Chem.**34**, 711-719, 1989, by N.Getoff: A review of the relationship between $Q(e_{aq}^{-})$ and Q_F of excited compounds in aqueous solution, with permission from Elsevier).

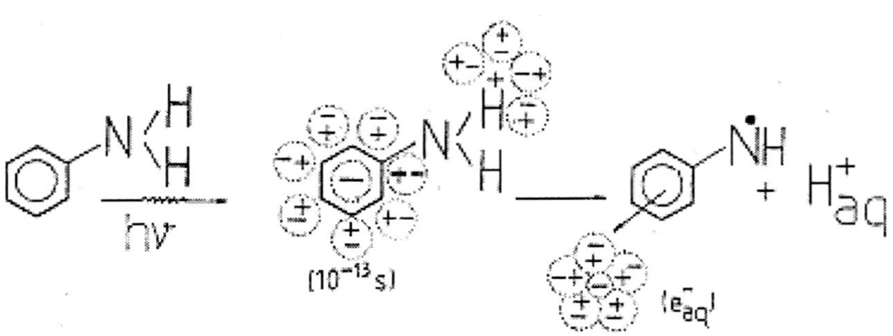

Figure 2.3.4. Schematic presentation of the electron ejection from aniline: formation of e_{aq}^{-}, H_{aq}^{+} and anilino radical, $C_6H_5NH^{\bullet}$ in aqueous solution. (Reprint from Radiat.Phys.Chem.**34**, 711-719, 1989, by N.Getoff: A review of the relation ship between $Q(e_{aq}^{-})$ and Q_F of excited compounds in aqueous solution, with permission from Elsevier).

As already mentioned trace elements play an important role as catalyst mediating biological processes of enzymes, hormones and various redox reactions in organism. The precise reaction mechanisms of these processes were, however, not yet elucidated.

2.4. Ozone Radicals

Ozone is formed not only in the upper atmosphere, but also on the earth surface, where above all the chlorophyll mediates its formation by solar energy from the oxygen, which is under normal conditions in triplet excited state ($^3O_2$). Ozone is a powerful oxidizing agent and by inhalation it can lead to harmful biological consequences, therefore it is of interest. Ozone decomposes in water at room temperature resulting in the formation of hydroperoxyl ($HO_2^\bullet$) and hydroxyl (OH) radicals, according to a chain reaction scheme early proposed by Weiss (1935) (see e.g. /10/):

Initiation:

$$O_3 + H_2O \longrightarrow HO_3^+ + OH^- \rightleftharpoons 2\,HO_2^\bullet \qquad (2.4.1)$$

$$O_3 + OH^- \longrightarrow HO_2^\bullet + O_2^{\bullet -} \qquad (2.4.2)$$

$$\longrightarrow OH + O_3^{\bullet -} \qquad (2.4.3)$$

$$HO_2^\bullet \rightleftharpoons H^+ + O_2^{\bullet -} \quad (pK = 4.8) \qquad (2.4.4)$$

Propagation:

$$O_3 + O_2^{\bullet -} + H^+ \longrightarrow OH + 2\,O_2 \qquad (2.4.5)$$

$$O_3 + OH \longrightarrow HO_2^\bullet + O_2 \qquad (2.4.6)$$

Termination: Combination of the radicals: OH, $HO_2^\bullet$ and $O_2^{\bullet -}$

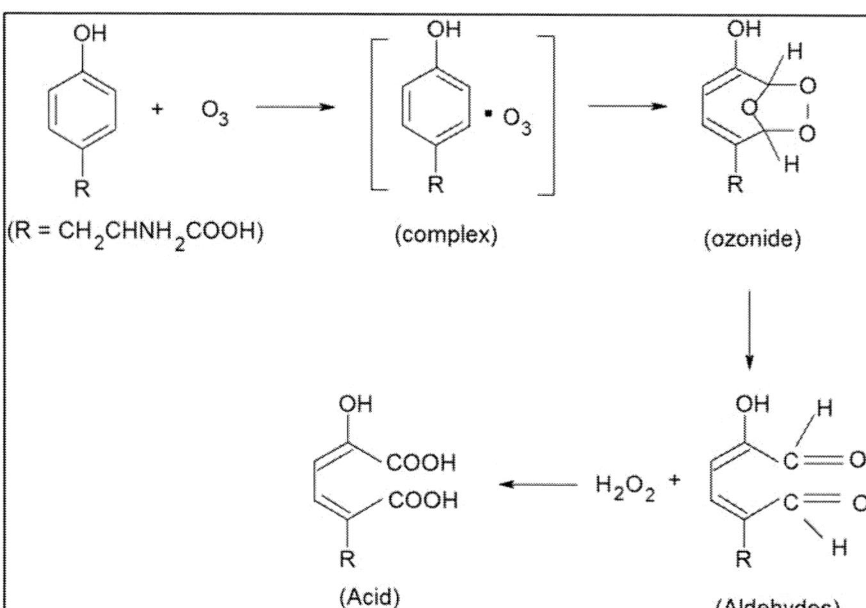

Scheme 2.4.1. Tyrosine decomposition by ozone

It should be mentioned that the free radicals generated in the human organism can also be strongly involved in the ozone decomposition. Thereby a number of oxidizing species are formed, which are attacking the cell components. The reactions involved in ozone degradation by oxidizing and reducing radicals, together with the corresponding reaction rate constants (k) are presented in Table 2.4.1. The data are resulting from pulse radiolysis studies, performed by various authors (for details see /11/)

It might be mentioned, that ozone attacks preferentially the double bonds of a compound, initiating the formation of various intermediates, which are leading to stable products. As an example the possible reaction of the tyrosine ozonation is shown on scheme 2.4.1.

The products shown in scheme 2.4.1. can be naturally further react with ozone on their double bonds. Hence, numerous of final products are formed. The ozone transients, such as OH, $HO_2^{\bullet}/O_2^{\bullet-}$, etc. (see Table 2.4.1) can react with components of the cells in organism leading to their destruction.

Table 2.4.1. Reactions and rate constants (k) of ozone decomposition in aqueous solution

Reaction		k (dm^3 mol^{-1} s^{-1})
$H + O_3 \longrightarrow HO_3^{\bullet}$		3.6×10^{10}
$e_{aq}^- + O_3 \longrightarrow O_3^{\bullet-}$		3.7×10^{10}
$HO_3 \overset{a}{\underset{b}{\rightleftharpoons}} H^+ + O_3^-$ ($pK_a = 8.2$)	(a)	$3.3 \times 10^{2\,a}$
	(b)	5.2×10^{10}
$O_3^{\bullet-} \overset{a}{\underset{b}{\rightleftharpoons}} O^{\bullet-} + O_2$	(a)	$3.3 \times 10^{3\,a}$
	(b)	3.0×10^9
$O_3^{\bullet-} + H^+ \longrightarrow OH + O_2$		9.0×10^{10}
$\quad \longrightarrow HO_3$		
$OH + O_3 \longrightarrow HO_2^{\bullet} + O_2$		1.1×10^8
$OH + O_3 \longrightarrow HO_4^{\bullet}$		2.0×10^9
$HO_4^{\bullet} \longrightarrow HO_2^{\bullet} + O_2$		$2.8 \times 10^{4\,a}$
$HO_4^{\bullet} + HO_4^{\bullet} \longrightarrow 2O_3 + H_2O_2$		5.0×10^9
$HO_4^{\bullet} + HO_3^{\bullet} \longrightarrow O_3 + H_2O_2 + O_2$		5.0×10^9
$OH + O_3^{\bullet-} + OH^- \longrightarrow 2O_2^{-\bullet} + H_2O$		8.5×10^8
$HO_2^{\bullet} + O_3 \longrightarrow H_2O_2 + O_2$		$< 10^4$
$\quad \longrightarrow OH + 2O_2$		
$O_2^{\bullet-} + O_3 \longrightarrow O_3^{\bullet-} + O_2$		1.6×10^9
$OH + HO_2^{\bullet} \longrightarrow O_2 + H_2O$		7.9×10^9
$HO_2^{\bullet} + HO_2^{\bullet} \longrightarrow H_2O_2 + O_2$		7.5×10^5
		3.7×10^6
$HO_2^{\bullet} + O_2^{\bullet-} \longrightarrow HO_2^{\bullet-} + O_2$		1×10^8
$O_2^{\bullet-} + O_2^{\bullet-} \longrightarrow O_2 + O_2^{2-}$		< 10
$O^{\bullet-} + HO_2^- \longrightarrow O_2^{\bullet-} + OH^-$		4×10^8

[a] Units in s^{-1}.

2. References

[1] Getoff N., 1967. Radiation Chemistry of Water, pp.273-309 in: "Radiation Chemistry (Fundamentals, Techniques, Applications) Eds. Kaindl, K. and Graul E.H., in German. Dr. Hüttig Publ.House, Heidelberg Germany.

[2] Spinks J.W.T. and Woods R.J., 1990. An Introduction to Radiation Chemistry. 3rd Edition, John Wiley and Sons, Inc.New York, Chichester, Toronto.

[3] Farhataziz and Rogers M.A.J., eds., 1978. Radiation Chemistry, Principals and Applications, VHC Publishers, Inc.New York, USA.

[4] Buxton G.V., Greenstock C.L., Helman W.P. and Ross A.B., 1988. Critical Review of Rate Constants for Reactions fo Hydrated Electrons, Hydrogen Atoms and Hydroxyl Radicals ($OH/O^{\bullet-}$) in Aqueous Solution. *J.Phys.Chem.Reference Data*, 17, 513-886.

[5] Calvert J.G. and Pitts Jr.J.N., 1966, Photochemistry, John Wiley and Sons, Inc. New York, London.

[6] Getoff N., 1968, Primary products of water photolysis at 1849 Å, Monatsh. Chem.99, 136-147.

[7] Getoff N., 1968, Vacuum-ultraviolet radiation; pp. 172-174 in "Radiation Chemistry and its application", Techn.Report Ser.No. 84, IAEA, Vienna, Austria.

[8] Getoff N. and Schenck G.O., 1968, Primary products of liquid water photolysis at 1236 Å, 1470 Å and 1849 Å, *Photochem.Photobiol.*8, 167-178.

[9] Getoff N., 1989. A review of the relationship between $Q(e_{aq}^-)$ and Q_F of excited compounds in aqueous solution. Radiat.Phys.Chem. 34, 711-719.

[10] Getoff, N., 2007, Anti-aging and aging factors in life. The role of free radicals, *Radiat.Phys.Chem.*76, 1577-1586.

[11] Getoff, N., 1977, Peroxyl radicals in the treatment of waste water solutions, pp. 483-506 in "Peroxyl Radicals", eds. z.B. Alfassi, John Wiley and sons Ltd., Chichester GB

Chapter 3

Measurement of Transients

Generally, there are presently several methods for the measurement of free radicals: pulse radiolysis, flash laser photolysis, electron spin resonance (ESR) and pulsed magnetic resonance (NMR) /see e.g. 1,2/. The frequently used ones in radiation chemistry and radiation biology is the pulse radiolysis technique because it offers some advantages. It allows the spectroscopic and kinetic characterization of transients, generated by reaction of the primary products of water radiolysis with e.g. given biological compound at each desired temperature. At higher temperatures the samples are irradiated in a special autoclave. For the sake of completeness of the subject matter, the pulse radiolysis method is briefly discussed.

3.1. Pulse Radiolysis Technique

This technique was developed in analogy to the flash photolysis method, where the initiating single light or laser short pulse was replaced by high energy electron pulse, usually 1 to 10 MeV /3-5/. It was first realized in England and USA in 1960. The method is based on the electron energy deposition e.g. in aqueous solution as very short single pulse (usually 10^{-6} to 10^{-12} s), provided by special designed electron accelerators. Principally, the duration of the electron pulse should be shorter than the life-time of the transients to be investigated in order to register their formation and decay.

For illustration, the pulse radiolysis equipment of the University of Vienna is presented briefly. Figure 3.1 shows schematically the assembly, implementing FEBETRON 708 electron accelerator, which provides two synchronized high-intensity electron pulses of 0.8 MeV and 3 ns duration /6/. Since the provided dose per single pulse is very high, it was reduced by metallic nets of fine mesh size. In order to obtain a desired dose per pulse (e.g. 10 Gy), several such nets were fixed together as an "electron beam filter", placed on both sides of the quartz cell. A certain part of the primary electron beam is also absorbed by the thermo-elements (T, Figure 3.1. B) and is registered on the two-channel oscilloscope as mV-value for each electron tube individually.

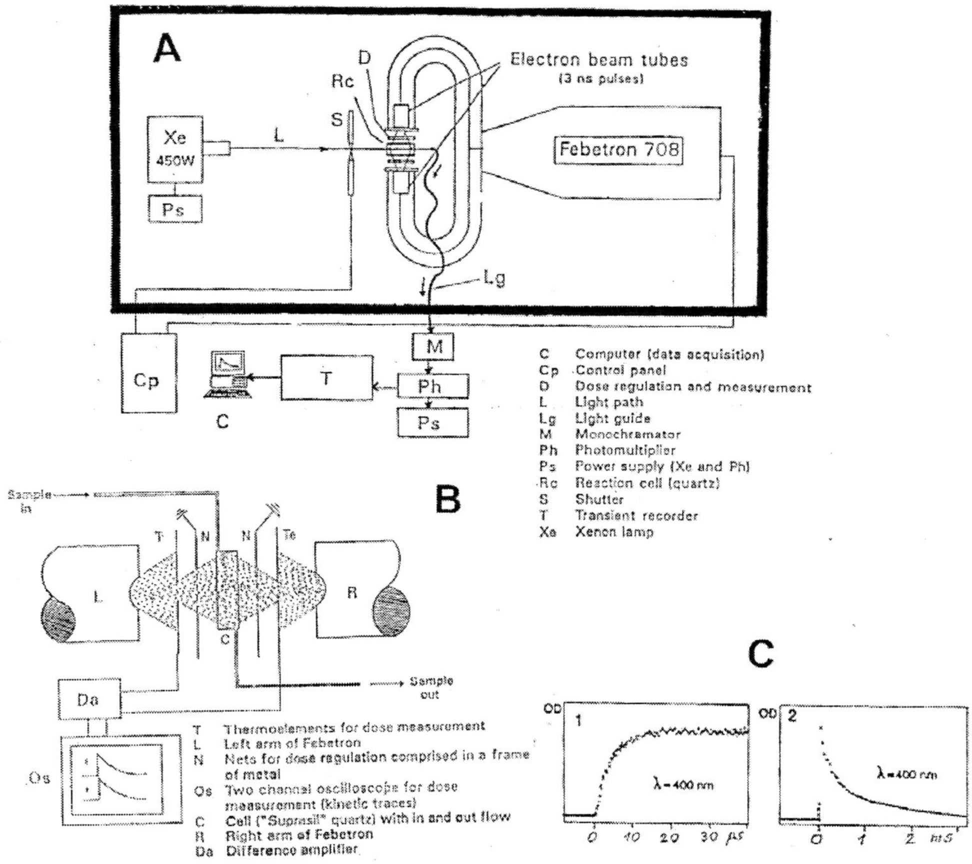

Figure 3.1. Pulse radiolysis equipment with FEBETRON 708, providing two synchronized electron pulses (0.8 MeV, 3 ns duration) at both sides of a quartz cell. (A) General view of the assembly. (B) Arrangement of thermoelements, "electron beam filter" and quartz cell between electron tubes. (C) kinetic traces : (1) formation and (2) decay of transients.(Reprinted from Nucl.Instr.Meth.Phys.Res.A 481, 81-85, 2002, by R.M.Quint and N.Getoff: Dose reduction and dose measurement for pulse radiolysis equipment, type Febetron 708, with permission from Elsevier).

The fraction of the electron beam, attenuated by the appropriate "electron beam filter" of both sides of the cell is penetrating nearly homogenously the solution, producing a homogenous distribution of radicals. The mV-values registered at the same time on the two channel oscilloscope are related to the absorbed radiation dose in the cell.

The calibration of the absorbed radiation dose (Gy) per single pulse is separately performed by a chemical dosimeter using various doses per pulse. The last ones are brought in relation by a calibration curve showing the dose/pulse (Gy) as a function of the corresponding mV-values registered by the oscilloscope. This method delivers an exact absorbed dose/pulse provided by each electron tube.

The focussed analyzing light (XBO 450 W xenon lamp, "Osram", equipped also for flashing operation) is passing first the quartz cell (before and after the electron pulse) and then the monochromator (M; Jobin Yvon) and the light of selected wavelength (nm) reaches the photomultiplier (Hamamatsu R955) and the amplified electrical impulse is registered at the transient recorder (Philips PM 3320) as a function of time as well as on a computer for data acquisition (Figure 3.1.). According to the adjustment on the transient recorder, the transient formation or decay, respectively, is registered (Figure 3.1. C1 and C2). From the course of the time profiles C1 and C2 the corresponding reaction rate constants are calculated. The absorption spectrum of corresponding transients can be obtained by determining the absorption (OD = optical density) for the light path of the cell at various wavelengths. The kinetic and spectroscopic evaluation procedure of such measurements is described in various essays (e.g. /4/). Nowadays, however, these calculations are performed automatically by computer on line, implementing appropriate computer programme.

In view of time saving the above described equipment for spectroscopic and kinetic measurements and acquisition of the data, can be replaced by a multiple-wavelength multi-time scale optical absorption system. Using such electronic equipment one can register the entire absorption spectrum at various times after the pulse end (e.g. ns) and the kinetics at each desired absorption maximum by implementing just one single electron pulse (see later, e.g. pulse radiolysis of β-carotene).

In order to study ultrafast chemical and radiation-induced biological reactions, picosecond time resolution pulse radiolysis systems with various modifications were developed (see e.g. /7-13/). Based on the ambition to register very early processes initiated by electron beam and stimulated by femtosecond pulsed laser in the past few years, a new type of pulse radiolysis equipment are generated. In the subpicosecond pulse radiolysis equipment, a powerful laser providing femtosecond pulses is triggering a photocathode of appropriate semiconductor, acting as electron source. The primary extracted electron pulse, having the same pulse length as the excitation laser pulse, is accordingly amplified and directed to the irradiation cell. The time synchronization of pulsed laser electron beam and a fast streak camera permit kinetic studies of species in femtosecond time range. Several laboratories in Japan, USA and Europe are operating such ultra-fast pulse radiolysis systems.

3. References

[1] Farhataziz and Rogers M.A.J., eds., 1978. *Radiation Chemistry, Principals and Applications*, VHC Publishers, Inc., Weinheim, Germany.

[2] Spinks J.W.T. and Woods R.J., 1990. *An Introduction to Radiation Chemistry. 3rd Edition,* John Wiley and Sons, Inc.New York, Chichester, Toronto.

[3] Keene J.P., 1965. Technique of pulse radiolysis by optical absorption; pp.1-14 in "*Pulse radiolysis*", eds. Ebert M., Keene J.P., Swallow A.J. and Baxendale J.H.; Academic Press, London, GB.

[4] Getoff N., 1969. Pulse radiolysis, theory of method and applications (in German), *Allgem.Prakt.Chem.* 20, 353-361.

[5] Paterson L.K., 1987. Instrumentation of measurements of transient behaviour in radiation chemistry, pp. 65-96 in "*Radiation Chemistry, Principals and Applications*", eds. Fahataziz and Rodgers M.A.J., VHC-Publishers, Inc. New York.

[6] Quint R.M. and Getoff N., 2002. Dose reduction and dose measurement for pulse radiolysis equipment, type FEBETRON 708, *Nucl.Instr.Meth.in Phys.Res.* A481, 81-85.

[7] Bronskill M.J., Taylor W.B., Wolf R.K. and Hunt J.W., 1970, Design and performance of a pulse radiolysis system capable of picosecond time resolution, *Rev.Sci.Instr.*41, 333-340.

[8] Jonah C.D., 1975, A wide-time range pulse radiolysis system of picosecond time resolution, *Rev.Sci.Instr.*46, 62-66.

[9] Kobayashi H. and Tabata Y., 1985, A 20 ps time resolved pulse radiolysis using two linacs, *Nucl.Instr.Methods* B 10/11, 1004-1006.

[10] Yoshida Y. Mizutani Y., Kozawa T., Saeki A., Saeki S., Tagawa S. and Ushida K., 2001, Development of laser synchronized picosecond pulse radiolysis systems, *Radiat. Phys.Chem.*6, 313-318.

[11] Wishard J.F., Cook A.R. and Miller J.R., 2004, The LEAF picosecond pulse radiolysis facility at Brookhaven National Laboratory, *Rev.Sci.Instrum.*75, 4359-4366.

[12] Kawguchi M., Ushida K., Kashiwagi S, Kuroda R., Kuribayashi T., Kobayashi M. Hama Y. and Washio M., 2005, Development of compact picosecond pulse radiolysis system, *Nucl.Instr.Meth.Phys.Res.*B, 236, 425-431.

[13] Maringnier J.-L., Waele V.de, Monard F., Gobert F., Larbre J.-P., Demarque A., Mostafavi M. and Beloni J., 2006, Time resolved spectroscopy at the picosecond laser-triggered electron accelerator ELYSE, *Radiat.Phys.Chem.*75, 1024-1033.

Chapter 4

Antitumor Compounds

4.1. General Remarks

Much effort has been done in the last decades in the development and testing of numerous antitumor drugs. Some of them proved to be very efficient and were successfully implemented in the chemo- as well as in the radiation-therapy. Simultaneously, the modern science made intense search for new and effective antitumor compounds obtained from plants, vegetables and fruits. In addition to this it has been succeeded e.g. to cultivate tomatoes with increased content on lycopen and broccoli on indol. The multisided preventive as well as curative effect of isoflavones and related substances is nowadays well founded and rapidly implemented. The research activities in this field became enormously and there is already an abundant literature in this field. It might be mentioned the multiple action of inositol, which is contained in various foods, e.g. peanuts, beans, rice, corn, sesame, sunflower seeds etc. Inositol is successfully used for prevention and treatment of cancer, osteoporosis, heart disease etc. (/1, 2/ and refs. therein). In the present treatise two cytostatica, mitomycin C and procarbacine were discussed as a model of studies.

4.2. Mitomycin C

Mitomycin C (MMC) is proven to be an efficient antitumor antibiotic against a number of human neoplasms, such as breast, lung, gastrointestinal, genitourinary, gynaecologic etc. tumors. It has been clinically implemented in Japan since 1950 and later on since about 1970 also in the USA, Europe and other countries in Asia /3,4/. MMC is isolated from *streptomyces caespitosus* and is primarily inactive, however, it can be activated practically in every kind of cells in the organism. Its peculiar chemical structure (aziridine, carbamate and quinoic cytotoxic groups on the same pyrrole nucleus, 1,2a-indolic) lend it preferential toxicity towards hypoxic cells. It is generally assumed that MMC has to be activated under anaerobic conditions either enzymatically by a proper electron donor (e.g. NADPH-cytochrome P-450 reductase; see e.g. /5/), chemically or by ionizing radiation /6-8/ in order to be converted into a quinone by one-electron reduction or to hydroquinone by two electron reduction process. It also has been observed, that using a high-dose MMC schedules, peroxyl radicals are formed, which can induce DNA-breaks and other processes /4/.

Although a great number of studies were carried out under various conditions, concerning the elucidation of the various MMC biological properties, its reaction mechanism appears to be still not completely understood. This can be demonstrated by the fact, that MMC can react not only with e_{aq}^- (formation of activated semiquinone of quinine /6-9/), but also with OH-radicals to result into MMC-OH adducts. The last ones add oxygen, generating MMC-peroxyl radicals, $(MMC.OH)O_2^{\bullet}$, /10,11/. It has been also shown that under appropriate media conditions MMC can react with H atoms /12/ and even eject or transfer one electron to an acceptor in order to convert into a radical cation, $MMC^{+\bullet}$ /13/. The spectroscopic and kinetic characteristics of the mentioned MMC-transients will be firstly presented and briefly discussed.

4.2.1. Mitomycin Transients

Reactivity of MMC with e_{aq}^-

As above indicated MMC can practically react with each type of free radicals generated in the organism, where the biological sequences of the resulting different MMC-species are far-reaching unknown. This fact could perhaps partly explain some side effects of this drug. For illustration and better understanding of the subject, some spectroscopic and kinetic data of the respective MMC-transients are briefly presented and discussed.

The cytostatic action of MMC is generally attributed to its reduced semiquinone form ($MMC^{\bullet-}$, radical anion), which is investigated by several research groups from different point of view, as mentioned above /5-9/.

The absorption spectrum of $MMC^{\bullet-}$ transients, reproduced for general information, is presented in Figure 4.2.1., where as insert the kinetic traces of some wavelengths are also given /9/. In the applied aqueous airfree medium 44% e_{aq}^-, 10% H and 46% OH radicals are operative, but OH and in part the H atoms are scavenged by the t-butanol. Hence, the remaining e_{aq}^- are the only acting species, producing $MMC^{\bullet-}$ radical anions:

$$MMC + e_{aq}^- \rightarrow MMC^{\bullet-} \quad (k = 2.2 \times 10^{10}\ L.mol^{-1}.s^{-1}) \qquad (4.1)$$

The spectrum of $MMC^{\bullet-}$ shows 15 μs after the 0.4 μs electron pulse two maxima in the UV-range and one at 510 nm ($\varepsilon = 10.000\ L.mol^{-1}.cm^{-1}$).

The kinetic traces (Figure 4.2.1., insert) show the formation of $MMC^{\bullet-}$ species, which is completed with 8-10 μs. Their decay in a time range upto 3 ms is, however, different. This indicates the existence of several MMC-transients, having distinct life times and decay constants, e.g. in the UV-range it is $k_1 = 2.1 \times 10^{3}\ s^{-1}$ (first order reaction) and at 510 nm (absorption maximum), $2k = 4.6 \times 10^{8}\ L.mol^{-1}.s^{-1}$ (second order reaction).

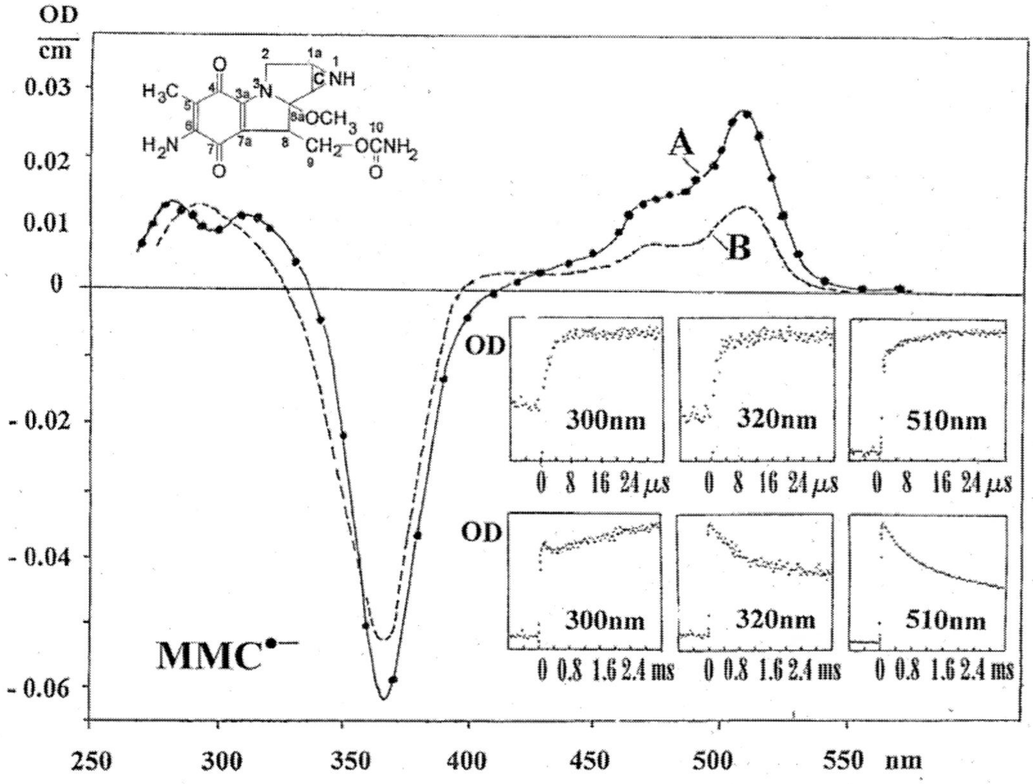

Figure 4.2.1. Transient absorption spectrum resulting form $3x10^{-5}$ mol/L MMC and 0.1 mol/L t-BuOH, pH 6.5 in airfree aqueous solution: (A) 15 μs after pulse end, (B) 3 ms after pulse end; OD/cm values normalized to 10 Gy. Insert: Kinetic traces at various wavelengths. (Reprinted from Radiat.Phys.Chem. 60, 351-358, 2001 by N.Getoff: Cytostatica efficiency enhancement by vitamins C, E and β-carotene under irradiation. State of the art, with permission from Elsevier).

The individual biological action of the produced MMC-radicals is presently not known. Generally, the reaction mechanism of the e_{aq}^- attack on MMC is based on the experiments by Pann et al. /5/ and Tomasz et al /6/, who isolated and identified the major covalent MMC-DNA adduct (Scheme 4.2.1.). Its build-up and existence explains ultimately the role of the $MMC^{\bullet-}$ species in the antitumor action of MMC, via the reaction with e_{aq}^- (eq. 4.1.).

However, no information exists about the biological action of the other MMC transients, generated by e_{aq}^- attack on the drug.

Reactivity of MMC with H Atoms

In order to demonstrate the many-sided reactivity of MMC and to point out the biological consequences of these processes, the attack of H- and OH-radicals, the effect of oxygen and the formation of MMC-radical cation ($MMC^{\bullet+}$) are very briefly reviewed. Although these data are published in the last few years they are very little known. Therefore, the biological fate of the above mentioned transients is generally not yet considered. Some data resulting from experiments in vitro (see later) just indicate their very important consequences by implementation.

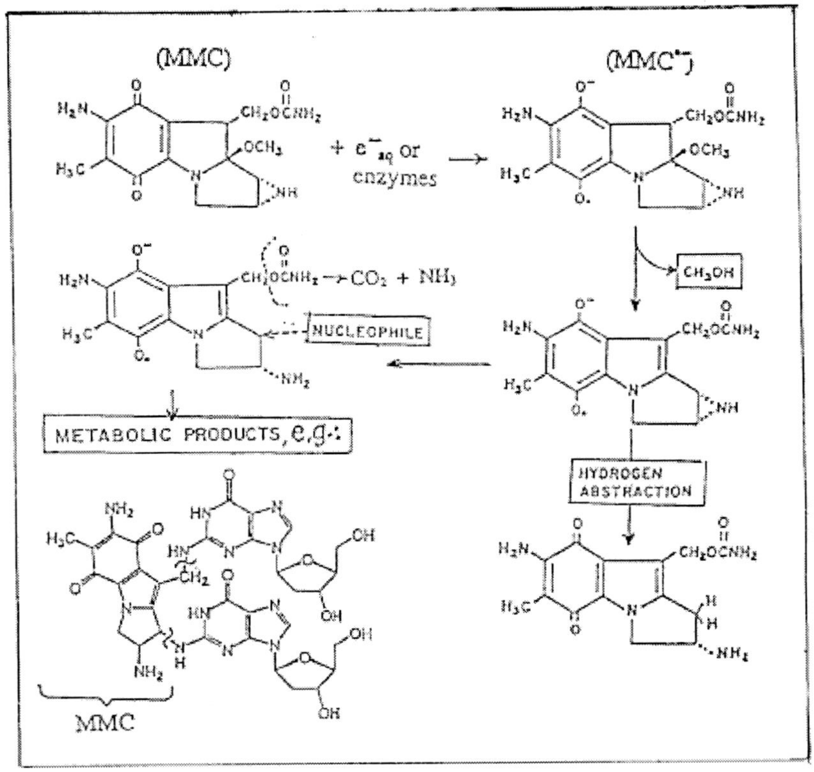

Scheme 4.2.1. Formation of $MMC^{\bullet-}$ radical anion and its subsequent reactions: elimination of methanol, cleavage of aziridine ring, formation of 2,7-diaminomitosene by hydrogen abstraction as well as cleavage of carbamate chain (build up of NH_3 and CO_2) and of various metabolic products (MMC-DNA adducts).

Some preliminary pulse radiolysis experiments were performed in the measurement of the *MMC-hydrogen adduct (MMC.H)*, using airfree, acid aqueous solution (pH ~ 2) as well as neutral media (pH ~ 7.4) /12/. As OH-scavenger tert-butanol was applied. Under these conditions the consumption of H-atoms by tert-butanol can be neglected.

$OH + t\text{-}C_4H_9OH \rightarrow t\text{-}C_4H_8OH^\bullet + H_2O$ ($k = 5.5\times10^{8}$ $L.mol^{-1}.s^{-1}$) (4.2)

$H + t\text{-}C_4H_9OH \rightarrow t\text{-}C_4H_8OH^\bullet + H_2$ ($k = 9\times10^{4}$ $L.mol^{-1}.s^{-1}$) (4.3)

$H + MMC \rightarrow MMC.H$ (H-adduct of MMC) (4.4)

(at pH = 2 is k ~ 9×10^{8} $L.mol^{-1}.s^{-1}$)

(at pH ~ 7.4 is k ~ 7×10^{7} $L.mol^{-1}.s^{-1}$)

The observed transient spectrum in acid media shows one sharp maximum at 250 nm (ε = 1.100 $L.mol^{-1}.cm^{-1}$) and an absorption band at 415 nm (ε = 250 $L.mol^{-1}.cm^{-1}$) in addition to a small one at 360 nm and a very weak absorption in the visible range. From the build-up kinetics at 250 nm and 415 nm absorption bands a mean value of the rate constants for the MMC.H formation in acid media is calculated as given above.

In neutral solution the MMC.H species have absorption maxima at 290 nm (ε = 160 $L.mol^{-1}.cm^{-1}$) and 500 nm (ε = 190 $L.mol^{-1}.cm^{-1}$) in addition to very weak absorptions at 420 nm and 610 nm. It is interesting to note, that in acid as well as in neutral solution a mixed decay kinetics has been observed. This indicates, that the H-atoms can attack the MMC molecule on various positions, leading to the formation of several types of MMC transients. About their biological properties presently nothing is known. It should be also noticed, that the H-species can to some extent also react with MMC by H-abstraction in addition to the adduct formation.

Reactivity of MMC with OH radicals

Since the OH radicals play a rather important role in the human organism, it was of special interest to learn about their reactivity towards MMC. With regard to the molecular structure of MMC it is expected, that the double bonds of the quinone ring will be preferable attacked by OH: *formation of OH-adducts: MMC.OH.* In addition to this process also H-abstraction from the –NH and $–NH_2$ groups, but less from the $–CH_3$ groups will take place. As a result, again various types of MMC-transients are expected. The situation is even more complicated in the presence of air, where e_{aq}^- and H are converted into peroxyl radicals (see Table 2.4.1. and Appendix). Simultaneously, O_2 is adding to the $MMC.OH^•$ adducts and other MMC-species resulting into unstable MMC-peroxyl radicals ($[MMC.OH]O_2^•$).

The transient absorption spectrum resulting from the OH-attack on MMC in aqueous neutral solution is presented in Figure 4.2.2. /10/. It is somewhat similar to that of $MMC^{•-}$ species, however, the kinetics are naturally different.

$$MMC + OH \rightarrow MMC.OH \quad \text{(OH-adducts)} \qquad (4.5a)$$

$$ \rightarrow MMC^• + H_2O \qquad (4.5b)$$

$$(\text{total } k = 5.8 \times 10^8 L.mol^{-1}.s^{-1})$$

The OH-reaction with MMC can take place on various positions on the molecule, hence, different OH-adducts as well as various $MMC^•$ radicals can be formed. This is also illustrated by the observed variable decay traces in ms-range, shown as insert in Figure 4.2.2. In reality a number of MMC transients are formed, but their spectra are strongly superimposed. Only two groups of them, short lived (spectrum A) and long-lived (spectrum B) have been registered by pulse radiolysis. The analysis of the decay kinetics at 295 nm and 505 nm were found to be complex: upto 150 μs the MMC-species disappear by a first order reaction, k_1= $8.5x10^2 s^{-1}$ (decomposition or/and reaction with water (hydrolysis) or with the starting molecule). However in the ms-range they are following a second order process (reaction between radicals)(2k = $1.3x10^8 L.mol^{-1}s^{-1}$) /10/.

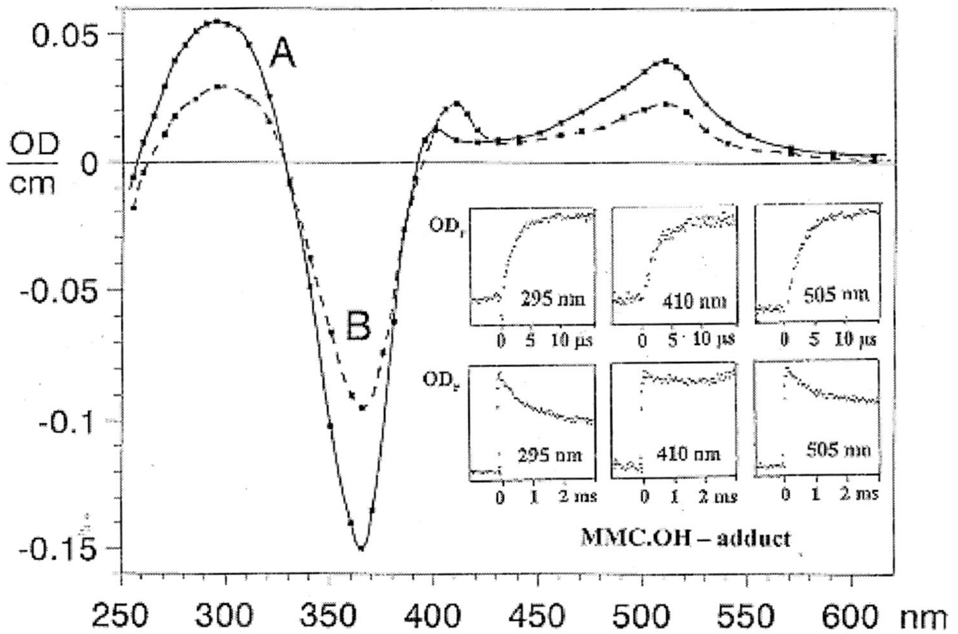

Figure 4.2.2. Transient absorption spectra resulting from OH-attack on aqueous $6x10^{-5}$ mol/L MMC saturated with N_2O (pH = 6.5) measured (A) 60 µs and (B) 3 ms after pulse end.*Insert:* Characteristic kinetic traces. (Reproduced from Radiat.Phys.Chem. 50, 575-583, 1997 by N.Getoff, S.Solar and R.M.Quint: One-electron oxidation of mitomycin C and its corresponding peroxyl radicals. A steady-state and pulse radiolysis study , with permission from Elsevier).

Peroxyl Radicals of MMC

The fate of the MMC-transients, as mentioned above, becomes even more complex in the presence of air, since: (i) oxygen is a strong competitor to MMC for e_{aq}^- and (ii) all radicals generated by the OH or/and H attack on MMC react with oxygen under formation of various MMC-peroxyl radicals:

$e_{aq}^- + O_2 \rightarrow O_2^{\bullet-}$ ($k = 1.9x10^{10}$ $L.mol^{-1}.s^{-1}$) (4.6.)

$e_{aq}^- + MMC \rightarrow MMC^{\bullet-}$ ($k = 2.2x10^{10}$ $L.mol^{-1}.s^{-1}$) (4.7.)

$MMC^{\bullet-} + O_2 \rightarrow MMC.O_2^{\bullet-}$ (peroxyl radical anion) (4.8.)

$MMC^{\bullet} + O_2 \rightarrow MMC.O_2^{\bullet}$ (peroxyl radical) (4.9.)

$(MMC.OH)^{\bullet} + O_2 \rightarrow (MMC..OH)O_2^{\bullet}$ (hydroxy-peroxyl radical) (4.10.)

The total absorption spectrum of the MMC-peroxyl radicals, measured in aqueous medium containing N_2O and O_2 in order to produce first MMC.OH and $MMC^{\bullet}$ species and subsequently to follow the addition of oxygen.

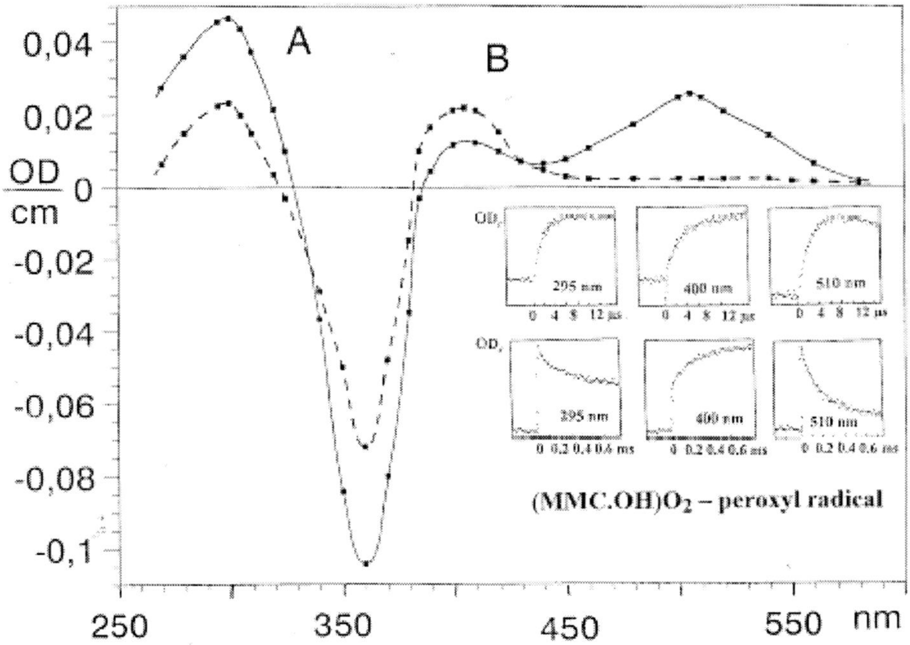

Figure 4.2.3. Transient absorption spectra obtained from OH-attack on aqueous $6x10^{-5}$ mol/L MMC in the presence of 80% N_2O and 20% O_2, pH = 6.5: (A) 12 μs and (B) 3.0 ms after pulse end. *Insert:* Characteristic kinetic traces. (Reproduced from Radiat.Phys.Chem. 50, 575-583, 1997 by N.Getoff, S.Solar and R.M.Quint: One-electron oxidation of mitomycin C and its corresponding peroxyl radicals. A steady-state and pulse radiolysis study , with permission from Elsevier).

The spectra are registered at 12 μs (A) and 3 ms after pulse (B) and are depicted in Figure 4.2.3. Spectrum (A) shows maxima at 290 nm (ε = 10.100 $L.mol^{-1}.cm^{-1}$), 410 nm (ε = 2.900 $L.mol^{-1}.cm^{-1}$) and 520 nm (ε = 5.500 $L.mol^{-1}.cm^{-1}$). The absorption maxima of spectrum (B) are naturally strongly reduced. Spectrum (A) is very similar to that of MMC.OH transients, however, with the exception of the differences between the formation and decay kinetics of both types of MMC species, given as insert in Figure 4.2.2. and 4.2.3.

The total rate constant for the O_2-addition on the MMC-species (eqs. 4.8. and 4.9.) was determined at pH = 6.5-9.5 to be k = $3x10^{8}$ $L.mol^{-1}.s^{-1}$). The peroxyl radicals decay according to a first order reaction, $k_1 = 7x10^{3}$ s^{-1} /10/.

Effect of Oxygen

As already indicated, both MMC and O_2 are competitors in respect to their reactivity with e_{aq}^- (eqs. 4.6. and 4.7.). Based on this fact and with regards to the biological role of $MMC^{\bullet-}$ transients in the formation of DNA-MMC adducts, stopping the multiplication of cancer cells, the effect of oxygen appeared to be of special interest. With special designed pulse radiolysis experiments using formate to convert OH and H into $^{\bullet}COO_2^-$ species, which are able to transfer one electron to MMC in airfree aqueous media, the highest yield of $MMC^{\bullet-}$ species are obtained (see also Chapter 3.1.)

$$HCOO^- + OH \rightarrow {}^{\bullet}CO_2^- + H_2O \ (k = 2.7x10^{9}\ L.mol^{-1}.s^{-1}) \qquad (4.11)$$

$$HCOO^- + H \rightarrow {}^{\bullet}CO_2^- + H_2 \ (k = 2.5x10^8 \ L.mol^{-1}.s^{-1}) \quad (4.12)$$

$${}^{\bullet}CO_2^- + MMC \rightarrow MMC^{\bullet -} + CO_2 \quad (4.13)$$

$$e_{aq}^- + MMC \rightarrow MMC^{\bullet -} \ (k = 2.2x10^{10} \ L.mol^{-1}.s^{-1}) \quad (4.14)$$

$$MMC^{\bullet -} + O_2 \rightarrow MMC + O_2^{\bullet -} \ (k = 2x10^9 \ L.mol^{-1}.s^{-1}) \quad (4.15)$$

By adding known amounts of oxygen to this media it was possible to observe the electron transfer from $MMC^{\bullet -}$ to O_2. This process is illustrated by the kinetic profiles shown in Figure 4.2.4 /10,11/. This is an important process, which can play an essential role in the cancer therapy implementing MMC as antitumor cytostaticum.

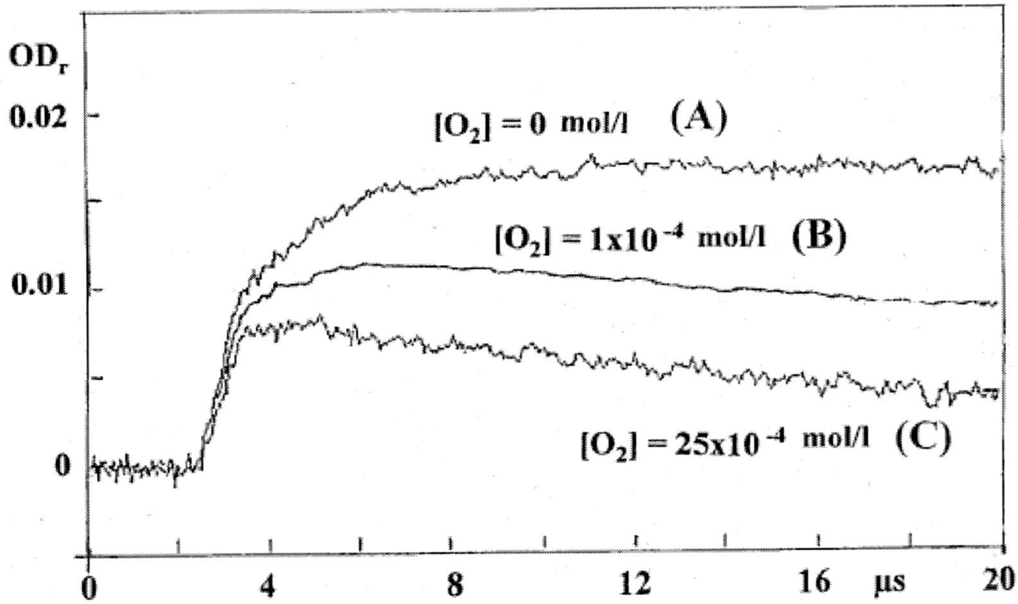

Figure 4.2.4. Electron transfer from $MMC^{\bullet -}$ species to O_2 studied by pulse radiolysis in aqueous solution (pH = 8.5) containing $3x10^{-4}$ mol/L MMC and 0.1 mol/L $HCOO^-$, saturated with argon (A); in the presence of $1x10^{-4}$ mol/L O_2 (B) and by adding of $25x10^{-4}$ mol/L O_2 (C). absorbed dose: 5.5 Gy per 0.1 µs electron pulse. (Reproduced from Radiat.Phys.Chem. 50, 575-583, 1997 by N.Getoff, S.Solar and R.M.Quint: One-electron oxidation of mitomycin D and its corresponding peroxyl radicals. A steady-state and pulse radiolysis study , with permission from Elsevier).

Mitomycin C Radical Cation

The investigations in this respect have been stimulated by some uncommon results obtained in experiments in vitro in aerated media in the presence of MMC (see later). The formation of MMC-radical cation ($MMC^{\bullet +}$) was observed by the attack of $Br_2^{\bullet}$ and $J_2^{\bullet -}$ species on MMC /12/.

More precise experiments were performed using $SO_4^{\bullet -}$ radicals as electron acceptor, produced simultaneously from persulfate ions by a single electron pulse in media containing MMC and t-butanol as OH-scavenger /13/. In this case MMC is acting as an electron donor:

$$MMC + SO_4^{\bullet -} \rightarrow MMC^{\bullet +} + SO_4^{2-} \qquad (4.16)$$

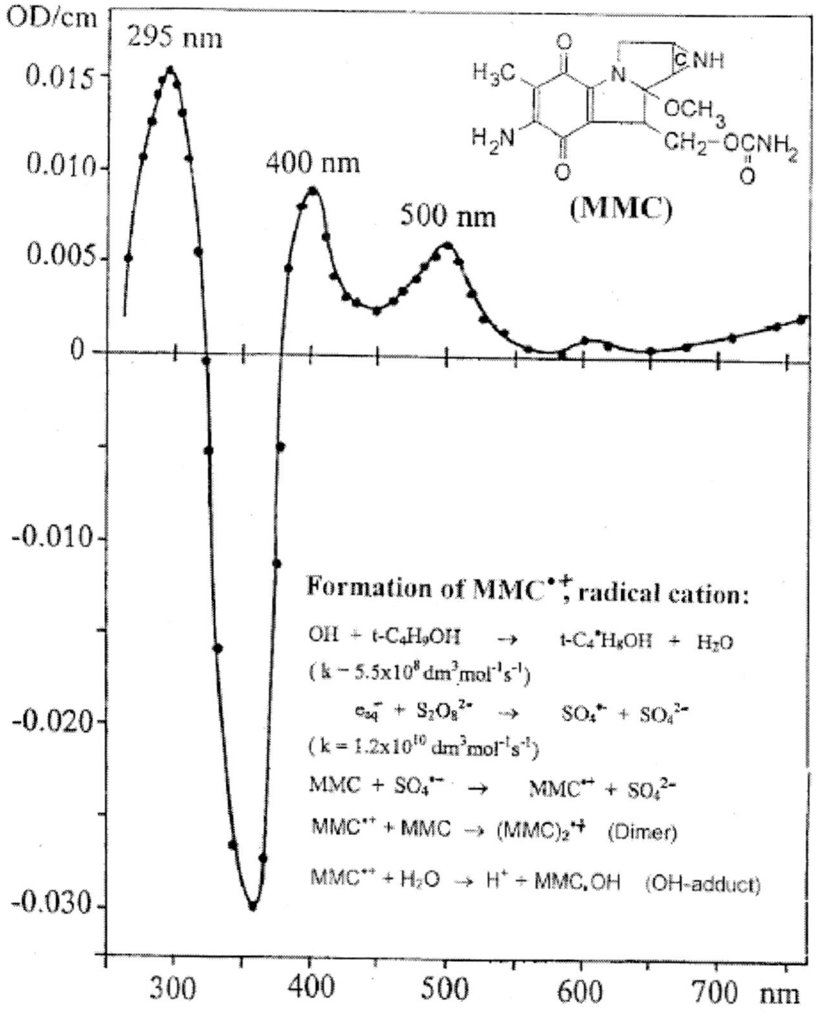

Figure 4.2.5. Absorption spectrum of $MMC^{\bullet +}$ species, observed 40 μs after 0.4 μs electron pulse in airfree aqueous medium: $6x10^{-6}$ mol/L MMC, $7x10^{-4}$ mol/L $S_2O_8^{2-}$ and $2x10^{-2}$ mol/L tert-butanol as OH scavenger (pH = 6.5). *Insert:* in the process involved reactions. (Reprinted from Int.J.In vivo **17**, 173-176, 2003 by N.Getoff: Mitomycin C radical cation studied by pulse radiolysis , with permission of the Journal). The degradation course of PC by various types of free radicals in aqueous media is shown in Figure.4.3.1.

The absorption spectrum of the generated $MMC^{\bullet +}$ species is shown in Figure 4.2.5. It has several maxima in the range of 300 nm upto 850 nm. The disappearance of $MMC^{\bullet +}$ transients was found to follow a second order reaction (eq. 4.17). However, these species can principally react with the starting compound forming dimers (eq. 4.18) or undergo hydrolysis resulting into MMC.OH-adduct (eq. 4.19).

$$2\,MMC^{\bullet +} \rightarrow \text{products} \quad (2k = 4.6x10^{9}\ L.mol^{-1}.s^{-1}) \qquad (4.17)$$

$MMC^{\bullet+} + MMC \rightarrow (MMC)_2^{\bullet+}$ (dimer) (4.18)

$MMC^{\bullet+} + H_2O \rightarrow H^+ + MMC.OH$ (adduct) (4.19)

The last two processes very likely proceed to a small fraction and therefore could not be registered.

The electron ejection from MMC, resulting into $MMC^{\bullet+}$ species in human organism can probably occur enzymatically, e.g. by the catalytic properties of cytochrome P-450. Very likely the $MMC^{\bullet+}$ radical cations will react specifically with macromolecular nucleotides and/or undergo other processes (e.g. according eqs. 4.18. and 4.19.), cleavage of the aziridine ring etc. resulting finally into metabolic products with DNA, as reported above for $MMC^{\bullet-}$ species. Further investigations are needed in this respect in order to elucidate the biological mechanism of $MMC^{\bullet+}$ transients.

4.3. Procarbacine

Procarbacine (N-(1-methylethyl)-4-[(2-methylhydrazino)-benzyl]benzamide; Natulan, Matulane, R0-4-6467) is frequently implemented in chemotherapy, as well as in combination with radiation therapy. It is used in the treatment of Hodgkin´s disease and lymphomas. However, its application is often accompanied by several side-effects, such as decrease of the immune system activity, generation of malignant tumors, cytotoxity with mitosis reduction etc. (see e.g. /14-16/).

Procarbacine (PC) is studied as a model compound in order to get a deeper insight in the reaction mechanisms about the action of oxidizing ($OH, O_2^{\bullet-}$) and reducing (e_{aq}^-,H) free radicals in such drugs. In addition to chemical analysis of products resulting by radiation–induced decomposition of PC, also experiments in vitro were performed /17/.

The most important data in this respect are briefly reported as an example for the combination of research methods in order to approach the real picture and better understanding of the involved mechanisms.

Depending on the actual environment and on the kind of radicals involved in the process, the formation of different products from PC was observed. In airfree media ammonia appears as a major radiolytic product in addition to a mixture of aldehydes. However, in aerated solutions the formation of carboxylic acids predominate in addition to a few not identified substances.

The highest degradation yield, G_i(-PC) = 5.60, was observed in solutions saturated with N_2O, where 90% OH and 10% H are involved in the process. In aerated media (acting species: 46% OH, 54% $O_2^{\bullet-}$) a G_i(-PC) = 3.45 was found, whereas in airfree solutions (44% e_{aq}^-, 46% OH, 10% H) the lowest G_i(-PC) = 2.85 was determined (insert in Figure 4.3.1.). Based on these data it is clear, that the OH radicals are the most powerful degradation radicals. As well known, these species are produced by oxidase enzyme in the liver, having a main function to decompose the consumed nutrients.

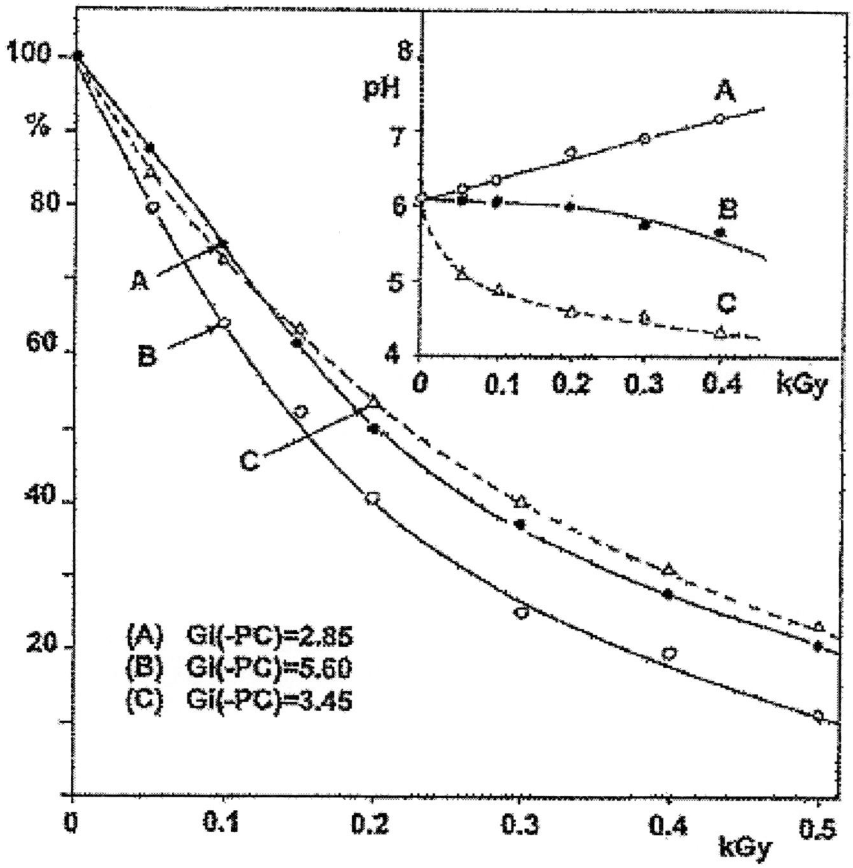

Figure 4.3.1. Free radical induced degradation of aqueous 10^{-4} mol/L PC (pH=4.6) saturated with: (A) Argon, (B) N_2O and (C) air as a function of absorbed radiation dose (kGy). *Insert:* pH-change in dependence of radiation dose (kGy) of the above solutions. (Reprinted from Anticancer Res. **24**, 1593-1596, 2004 by A.Delipetar-Grudl and N.Getoff: Procarbacine radiolysis and experiments in vitro, with permission of the Journal).

Experiments in vitro (model: Escherichia coli bacteria AB1157) showed that PC has in airfree (action of 44% e_{aq}^-, 10% H, 46% OH) as well as in aerated media (46% OH, 54% $O_2^{\bullet -}$) a rather well pronounced antitumor property, depending on the substrate concentration. However, in media saturated with N_2O (acting species: 90% OH, 10% H) PC proved to act as a potent radiation protecting substance (Table 4.3.1).

These results demonstrate on the one side the rather complicated radiation-induced reaction mechanism, but on the other hand, the role of the involved free radicals and of the above mentioned radiolytic products, which certainly are active involved in the actual biological processes in the presence of PC.

Table 4.3.1. ΔD_{37}(Gy)-values, derived from survival curves (model: Escherichia coli bacteria, AB 1157) taken as a function of absorbed dose (Gy), proportional to free radical concentration

PC (mol/L)	ΔD_{37}(Gy)-values[*)]		
	Airfree 44% e_{aq}^-,10% H,46% OH	Aerated 46% OH, 54% $O_2^{\bullet -}$	N_2O 10% H, 90% OH
0	0	0	0
10^{-4}	- 30	- 30	30
10^{-3}	- 65	- 50	10

*) ΔD_{37}(Gy)-value: D_{37}(Gy) is the Gy-value corresponding to $0.37N/N_0$-ratio The ΔD_{37}(Gy) is calculated by subtracting D_{37}-buffer value from the individual sample D_{37}-data; e.g.: D_{37}(sample)-D_{37}(buffer) = ΔD_{37}(Gy). The positive ΔD_{37}(Gy) values indicate radiation protecting ability and the negative ones, show the cytostatic efficiency of the system.

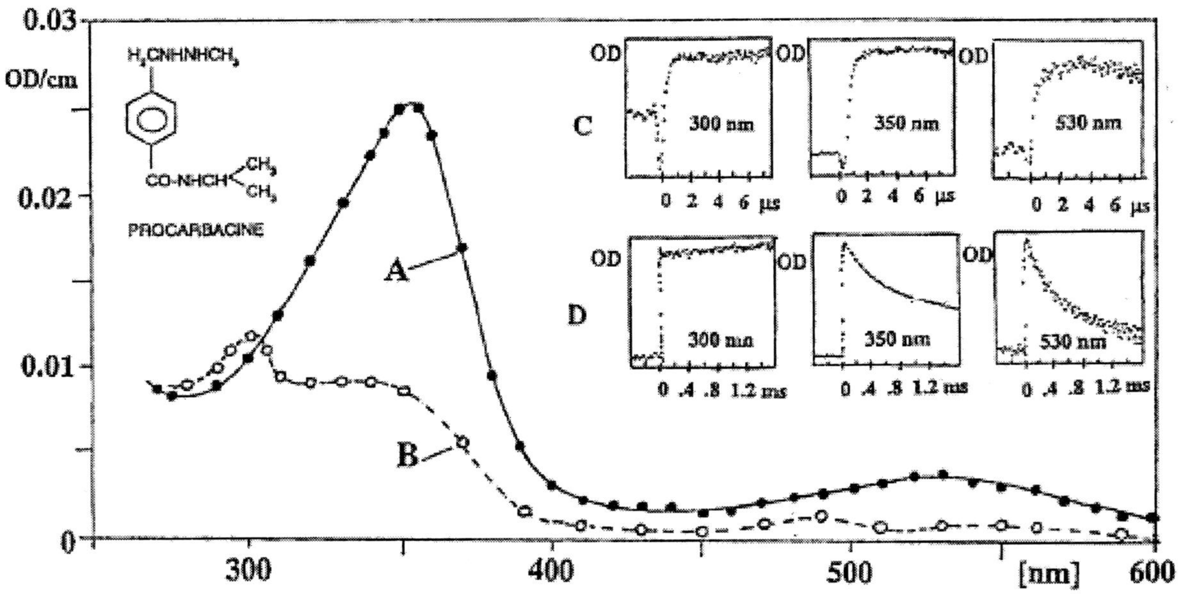

Figure 4.3.2. Total transient absorption spectra resulting from the reaction of OH radicals with PC. Solution: 5 x 10^{-5} mol/L PC, pH = 8.5, saturated with N_2O. Spectrum (A): 3.3 µs after pulse and (B) 1.5 ms after pulse. *Insert*: Kinetic profiles for formation (C) and decay (D) for the transients at different wavelengths.(Reprinted from Anticancer Res. 26, 405-410, 2006 by A.Delipetar-Grudl, S.Solar and N.Getoff: Reactions of OH-radicals with procarbazine. A pulse radiolysis and computer simulation study, with permission of the Journal).

Procarbacine Transients

In order to get a better understanding of the PC action mechanisms, the knowledge of its transients is needed. Hence, some recent pulse radiolysis and simulation computations were taken into consideration /18/. Studying the specific reactions of OH radicals as the most active species in aqueous PC solutions, the formation of two transients was registered: (A) measured 3 µs after 0.4 µs electron pulse (ε_{350} = 4,46x10^3 L.mol^{-1}.cm^{-1}) and (B) observed

1,5 ms after pulse end (Figure 4.3.2). The formation and decay kinetics, given as insert in Figure 4.3.1 show different courses, which indicate the existence of more than two transients.

The overall rate constant of the OH-attack on PC (eq. 4.20) as well as that for the H-atom (eq. 4.21) are given for information /18/.

$$OH + PC \rightarrow PC.OH\text{-transients} \quad (4.20)$$

(at pH~7: $k=3.7\times10^{9}\ L.mol^{-1}.s^{-1}$)

These radicals disappear in the absorption range of 500 to 600 nm by a first order reaction, $k = 1.75\times10^{3}\ s^{-1}$, likely forming dimers or/and react with water.

$$H + PC \rightarrow PC.H\text{-transients} \quad (4.21)$$

(at pH=2: $k=6.4\times10^{8}\ L.mol^{-1}.s^{-1}$)

Both, OH and H can attack the PC-molecule on various positions, resulting in various PC-transients. This fact initiated computer-simulation studies. The regioselectivity of the OH attack is related to the PC electron density, steric hindrance and to the stability of formed PC-transients. Based on these premises computations concerning the charge distribution of the optimized ground state PC molecule as well as of total energies and the formation enthalpies of the PC-possible radicals have been performed /18/. The transient absorption spectra registered by pulse radiolysis at 3.3 μs (A) and 1.5 ms (B) as well as some characteristic kinetic traces are shown in Figure 4.3.2. For illustration of the subject matter, the computed charge distribution of PC is presented in Figure 4.3.3.

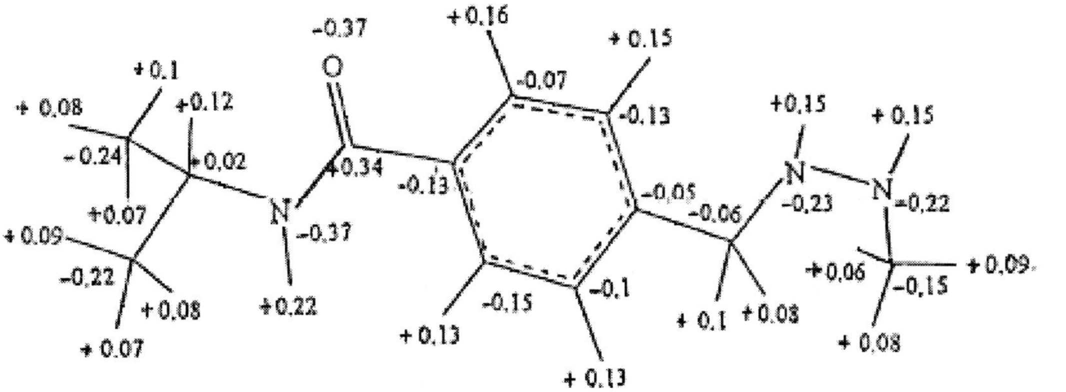

Figure 4.3.3. Charge distribution of the geometrically optimized procarbacine molecule. (Reproduced from Anticancer Res. 26, 405-410, 2006 by A.Delipetar-Grudl, S.Solar and N.Getoff: Reactions of OH-radicals with procarbazine. A pulse radiolysis and computer simulation study, with permission of the Journal).

The negative charges (Figure 4.3.3) show the following distribution: 33% are on N-atoms, 27% on C-atoms of the side chains, 25% on the aromatic ring carbons and the remaining 15% are on the oxygen atom. Outgoing from these data it is theoretically very likely to expect the formation of 9 different PC-radicals. The calculation of the formation enthalpies (ΔH_F) of the expected PC-species resulting from the OH-attack proves that spectrum (A), Figure 4.3.2 should correspond to OH-adduct on the ring position 6, because it has the highest negative formation enthalpy (-21.4 kJ/mol). Hence, it is stable enough to be measured. This species are followed by adduct formation on the ring-positions 3 and 2, respectively. They could not be individually registered, because they were superimposed. The three OH-adducts of PC are of biological importance.

The reviewed studies on PC demonstrate, that by combination of appropriate research methods (experiments in vitro, chemical analysis of radiolytic products, pulse radiolysis, computer simulations etc.) one can gain a more clear picture about reaction mechanisms. Such data can also explain undesired side effects of a given drug and help to optimize treatment procedure.

4. References

[1] Grases F., Simonet B.M., Vucenic I., Perelló J., Prieto R.M. and Shamsudin A.M., 2002, Effects of exogenous inositol hexaphosphate (Ins P6) on inositol triphosphate (Ins P3) and Ins P3 in malignant cells, tissues and biological fluids, *Life Sciences* 71, 1535-1546.

[2] Vanderlinden N.D. and Vucenik I., 2004, To good to be true?, Bearing Marketing Comm.Ltd., Mississanga ON., USA.

[3] Ogawa M., Rozencweig M., and Staquet M.J., (eds), 1982, Mitomycin C, Current Impact on Cancer Chemotherapy, Proceed.3rd Symp.pm New Drugs in Cancer Therapy, Brussels, Oct. 1981, Excerpta Medica, Amsterdam, Geneva, Tokyo.

[4] Taguchi T. and Aigner K.R., (eds.), 1991, Mitomycin C in Cancer Therapy Today; Proceed.15th Symp.Int.Cancer Congress, Hamburg, Germany 1990, Experta Medica, Amsterdam, Tokyo.

[5] Pann S.S., Andrews P.A., Glover C.J. and Bachur N.R., 1984, Reductive oxidation of mitomycin C metabolites catalyzed by NADPH-cytochrome P-450 reductase and xanthine oxidase., *J.Biology and Chemistry* 259, 956-966.

[6] Tomasz M., Chowdary D., Lipman R., Shimotakahara S., Veiro D., Walker V. and Verdine G.L., 1986, Reaction of DNA with chemically or enhymatically activated mitomycin C; Isolation and structure of the major covalent adduct. *Proceed.Nation.Acad. of Sci. USA* 83, 6702-6706.

[7] Butler J., Hoey B.M. and Swallow A.J., 1985, Reactions of semiquinone free radicals of anti-tumor agents with oxygen and iron complexes. FEBS 182, 95-98.

[8] Machtalere G., Honee-Levin Ch., Gardes A.M., Ferradini Ch. and Hickels B.; 1988, Pulse radiolysis study of the reduction mechanism of anti-tumor antibiotic mitomycin C; C.R.*Acad.Sci Paris,* 307, 17-22.

[9] Getoff N., 2001, Cytostatica efficiency enhancement by vitamins C, E and β-carotene under irradiation. State of the art, *Radiat.Phys.Chem.*60, 351-358.

[10] Getoff N., Solar S. and Quint R.M., 1997, One-electron oxidation of mitomycin C and its corresponding peroxyl radicals. A steady-state and pulse radiolysis study, *Radiat.Phys.Chem.*50, 575-583.

[11] Getoff N., 2002, Effect of antioxidants and oxygen in radiotherapy, Proceed.7th Int.Meet.Progress in Radio-Oncology, pp. 99-105; eds. Kogelnik H.D., Lukas P. and Sedelmayer F., Salzburg, Austria.

[12] Getoff N., 2000, unpublished results

[13] Getoff N., 2003, Mitomycin C radical cation studied by pulse radiolysis, *In vivo* 17, 173-176.

[14] Reuss K., Engert A., Tesch H. and Diehl V., 1996, Current clinical trails in Hodgkins disease, *Ann.Oncol.*7 (Suppl.4), 104-113.

[15] Schelong G., 1996, Treatment of children and adolescents with Hodgkins disease. The experience of the German-Austrian paediatric study group, *Bailliere's Clin.Haematol.*9, 619-634.

[16] Gundersen S., Lote K. and Wante K., 1998, A retrospective study of the value of chemotherapy as adjuvant therapy to surgery and radiotherapy in 3 and 4 gliomas, *Eur.J.Cancer* 34, 1565-1569.

[17] Delipetar-Grudl A. and Getoff N., 2004, Procarbacine radiolysis and experiments in vitro, *Anticancer Res.*24, 1593-1596.

[18] Delipetar-Grudl A., Solar S. and Getoff N., 2006, Reactions of OH-radicals with procarbazine. A pulse radiolysis and computer simulation study, *Anticancer Res.*26, 405-410.

Chapter 5

Antioxidant Vitamins

The water soluble vitamins: C,E and β-carotene are discussed as representative antioxidant compounds (acting as electron donors). There is an abundant literature covering their multiple biological properties and their very important role as supplementary nutrients needed for the health /1/. The presented discussion, however, concerns in general less known spectroscopic and kinetic characteristics, of their transients, generated by irradiation in aqueous media. These are namely the basis for understanding of the reaction mechanisms of their action. The same vitamin transients can be formed in the human organism likewise. As it will be shown, these species play a very essential role not only in the daily life, but also in connection with using drugs as well as by radiation treatment of patients.

5.1. Vitamin C (Ascorbic Acid)

The most investigated antioxidant vitamin, having a rather broad spectrum of biological properties, is the ascorbic acid (AH_2). In aqueous solution it has: $pK_1 = 4.3$ and $pK_2 = 11.8$, where the ascorbate (AH^-) in neutral media exists in two tautomeric forms. The ascorbate radicals have been studied from various points of view by pulse radiolysis /e.g. 2-6/ as well as by ESR method /7/. It has been established, that the OH radicals attack preferentially the double bonds, forming OH-adducts, and less the chain of ascorbate molecule.

In order to get a better insight of the subject matter, two series of pulse radiolysis experiments have been performed /8/. Series (A) using aqueous ascorbate (AH^-) solutions saturated with N_2O (conversion of e_{aq}^- into $OH^\bullet$, see eqs. 5.1 and 5.2) and series (B), where to solution (A) azide ion (N_3^-) was added. In this case the resulting $N_3^\bullet$ radicals specifically abstract one electron from AH^- molecule, forming ascorbate radical, $AH^\bullet$ (see reactions 5.3 to 5.5).

Series A:

$$AH + OH \rightarrow AHOH^{\bullet} \quad \text{(OH-adducts)} \qquad (5.1)$$

$$AH + OH \rightarrow H_2O + \text{various ascorbate species, under them aslo } AH^{\bullet} \qquad (5.2)$$

Series B:

$$e_{aq}^{-} + N_2O \rightarrow OH + OH^{-} + N_2 \qquad (5.3)$$

$$N_3^{-} + OH \rightarrow N_3^{\bullet} + OH^{-} \qquad (5.4)$$

$$N_3^{\bullet} + AH^{-} \rightarrow N_3^{-} + AH^{\bullet} \qquad (5.5)$$

$$2\,AH^{\bullet} \rightarrow AH_2 + DHA \qquad (5.6)$$

The ascorbate radical ($AH^{\bullet}$) disappears by disproportion (eq.5.6), resulting in ascorbate and dihydroascorbate (DHA).

In order to get only the reaction sequence (5.3) to (5.5), their reaction probability was calculated by considering the substrate concentrations and the corresponding reaction rate constants /8,9/.

The total absorption spectrum (A) obtained by reaction of OH radicals with ascorbate as well as the spectrum, (B) corresponding specifically to $AH^{\bullet}$ are depicted in Figure 5.1.1. The ascorbate radical, $AH^{\bullet}$, is most probably that kind of Vit.C transient, which is generated in the organism by electron transfer process (Vit.C action as electron donor).

Spectrum (A) has two maxima, a small one at about 300 nm and a sharp one at 360 nm as well as a broad absorption band from 400 to 600 nm, whereas the last one is not observed in spectrum (B). Based on these facts and on the corresponding kinetic data it is expected that the OH radicals can also generate $AH^{\bullet}$ transients according to eq. 5.7:

$$AH^{-} + OH \rightarrow AH^{\bullet} + OH^{-} \qquad (5.7)$$

Similar conclusion can also be derived from the spectroscopic and kinetic data given in Table 5.1.

Table 5.1. Spectroscopic and kinetic data of transients produced by OH attack on ascorbate (AH^{-}), corresponding to spectrum (A) and electron transfer form AH^{-} to $N_3^{\bullet}$ species, spectrum (B), respectively

Transient spectrum	λ_{max} [nm]	ε_{max} [L.mol^{-1}cm^{-1}]	Rate constant [L.mol^{-1}s^{-1}]	
			Formation	Decay
A	300	2.000	3.1×10^{9}	9.0×10^{5}
	360	3.240	6.5×10^{9}	7.1×10^{6}
	550	100	1.1×10^{8}	6.9×10^{7}
B	360	3.40	3.2×10^{9}	1.7×10^{7}

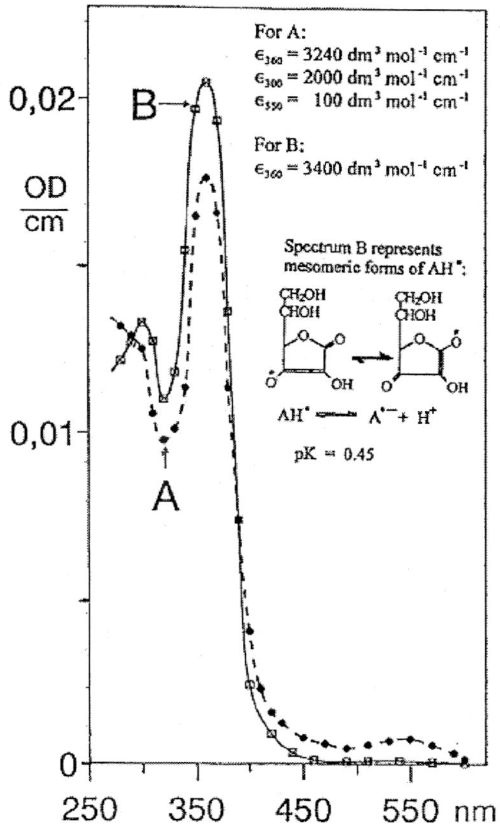

Figure 5.1.1. Transient absorption spectra resulting from the reaction of vit.C with OH radicals at pH = 8.4 (A) and with $N_3^{\bullet}$ species at pH = 7 (B). OD/cm-values normalized to 10 Gy. Insert: ε-values and mesomeric forms of vit.C radical. (Reprinted from Radiat.Phys.Chem.**60**, 351-358, 2001 by N.Getoff: Cytostatica efficiency enhancement by vitamin C, E and β-carotene under irradiation. State of the art; with permission from Elsevier)

From the results presented in Table 5.1 is obvious, that spectrum (A) is superimposed, representing several transients, most likely having different biological properties. Spectrum (B), however corresponds exclusively to the $AH^{\bullet}$ species, generated by vitamin C antioxidant action as electron donor.

5.2. Vitamin E (α-Tocopherol)

α-Tocopherol (Vitamin E, Vit.E; 2,5,7,8-tetramethyl-2-(4´,8´,12´-trimethyl-triecy)-6-chromanol) is practically unsoluble in water, but in organic solvents. It is a versatile antioxidant, which also protects cellular membranes against peroxidation by acting as a chain-breaking agent. Using ns-laser flash photolysis a strong absorption band in the range of 420 – 430 nm for the tocopheroxyl radical has been reported /10/. Later on it was of biological interest to establish the transients from Vit.E formed as a sequence of its antioxidant action, namely after its ejection of one electron. For this purpose pulse radiolysis experiments were performed using oxygenated dimethylsulfoxide (DMSO) as a solvent. In this case $G(e_s^-)$ =

G(DMSO$^{\bullet+}$) = 1.8 /11,12/. Under these experimental conditions Vit.E is involved in the following reactions (eq.5.8 – eq.5.13):

$$\text{DMSO} \rightsquigarrow \text{DMSO}^{\bullet+} + e_s^- + \text{species with small yields} \quad (5.8)$$

$$O_2 + e_s^- \rightarrow O_2^{\bullet-} \text{ (peroxyl radicals)} \quad (5.9)$$

$$\text{DMSO}^{\bullet+} + \text{Vit.E} \rightarrow \text{DMSO} + \text{Vit.E}^{\bullet+} \text{ (radical cation)} \quad (5.10)$$

$(k = 1 \times 10^9 \text{ L.mol}^{-1}.\text{s}^{-1})$

The produced radical cations (Vit.E$^{\bullet+}$) disappears mostly by radical-radical-reactions (eq.5.11), but to small extent also by first order mixed kinetics (eqs. 5.12 and 4.13).

$$k\,[\text{Vit.E}^{+\bullet} + R^{\bullet} \text{ (various species)}] = 4.7 \times 10^8 \text{ L.mol}^{-1}.\text{s}^{-1} \quad (5.11)$$

$$\text{Vit.E}^{\bullet+} + H_2O \rightarrow H^+ + + \text{Vit.E.OH (OH-adducts)} \quad (5.12)$$

$$2\ \text{Vit.E}^{\bullet+} \rightarrow \text{unknown products} \quad (5.13)$$

It is clear that the complete reaction mechanism of the Vit.E$^{\bullet+}$ species is not yet elucidated. Therefore, in the further considerations about the biological fate only Vit.E$^{\bullet+}$ transients are taken into account.

The absorption spectrum of Vit.E$^{\bullet+}$ radical cations is shown in Figure 5.2.1.

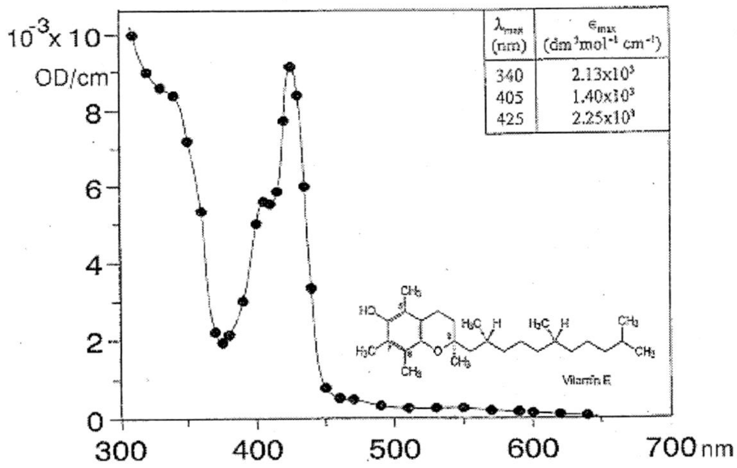

Figure 5.2.1. Transient absorption spectrum of vit.E$^{\bullet+}$ (5μs after 0.4 μs electron pulse resulting from 9.3 x 10^{-4} mol/L α-tocopherol in aerated DMSO solution (OD-values normalized to 10 Gy). Insert: Spectroscopic data. (Reprinted from Radiat.Phys.Chem.**55**, 699-704, 1999 by N.Getoff, I.Platzer and C.Winckelbauer: Transients and cooperative action of β-carotene, vitamin E and C in biological systems in vitro under irradiation; with permission from Elsevier).

The spectrum shows an absorption band in the range > 300 nm, in addition to a strong absorption maximum at 425 nm with a shoulder at 405 nm as well as very weak absorption in the range of 450 nm upto 650 nm. This indicates the existence of several structure forms of $Vit.E^{\bullet +}$ species.

It might be mentioned that the formation of vitamin E-acetate radical cation ($Vit.E\text{-}ac^{\bullet +}$) in oxygenated DMSO solution shows several maxima in the range of 300 upto 560 nm formed with $k = 8 \times 10^{8}$ $L.mol^{-1}.s^{-1}$, and disappears by first order reaction ($k_1 = 6 \times 10^{3}$ s^{-1}), very likely resulting into a dimer-cation $(Vit.E\text{-}ac)_2^{\bullet +}$ /9/.

It is of interest to note that Vit.E is also able to react with e_{aq}^{-} under special experimental conditions. This fact is of biological importance and shows its rather broad action domain. A preliminary rate constant for this reaction: $k(Vit.E + e_{aq}^{-} \rightarrow Vit.E^{\bullet -}) \sim 8.1 \times 10^{8}$ $L.mol^{-1}.s^{-1}$ was determined by pulse radiolysis method with a mixture of 90% ethanol and 10% water /13/.

5.3. β-Carotene

Naturally occurring are presently about 600 carotenoids characterized, of which about 10%, including β-carotene, are precursors of vitamin A (retinol). The most important of them, β-carotene (β-car) is provitamin A. It is widely distributed in the plant and animal kingdom and belongs like Vit.E to the group of "fat-soluble" vitamins. It can quench singulet oxygen and act as electron donor in tissues, especially at low oxygen tension, and is able to stimulate the immune response /1/.

In early pulse radiolysis studies the formation of all trans-β-carotene radical anion ($\beta\text{-car}^{\bullet -}$) is reported, having an absorption maximum, $\lambda_{max} = 880$ nm ($\varepsilon = 4.42 \times 10^{5}$ $L.mol^{-1}.cm^{-1}$) in n-hexane, and $\lambda_{max} = 900$ nm ($\varepsilon = 3.24 \times 10^{5}$ $L.mol^{-1}.cm^{-1}$) in cyclohexane /14/. The same authors observed absorption maxima of $\beta\text{-car}^{\bullet +}$ (radical cation) at 1040 nm ($\varepsilon = 2.15 \times 10^{5}$ $L.mol^{-1}.cm^{-1}$) and at 1050 nm ($\varepsilon = 2.02 \times 10^{5}$ $L.mol^{-1}.cm^{-1}$) in hexane and cyclohexane respectively. By conductivity measurements (10^{-5} mol/L β-car) in airfree hexane a rate constant for the formation of $\beta\text{-car}^{\bullet -}$ was determined, $k = 1.4 \times 10^{12}$ $L.mol^{-1}.s^{-1}$, as well as for $\beta\text{-car}^{\bullet +}$ species absorbing at 1050 in cyclohexane, $k = 1.1 \times 10^{11}$ $L.mol^{-1}.s^{-1}$ was measured. Both radical ions, $\beta\text{-car}^{\bullet -}$ at 880 nm and $\beta\text{-car}^{\bullet +}$ at 1040 nm in n-hexane were found to decay by second order reaction: $k(880\ nm) = 6.5 \times 10^{11}$ $L.mol^{-1}.s^{-1}$ and $k(1040\ nm) = 4.7 \times 10^{11}$ $L.mol^{-1}.s^{-1}$, respectively.

The formation of $\beta\text{-car}^{\bullet -}$ produced by pulse radiolysis of aqueous non-ionic micellar solution of TritonX-100 has also been observed at 865 nm ($k \sim 2 \times 10^{8}$ $L.mol^{-1}.s^{-1}$) /15/. The absorption characteristics of radical ions in various solvents have been subject of investigations from various points of view /16-18/.

Finally, the formation of β-carotene radical anion ($\beta\text{-car}^{\bullet -}$) species, registered by pulse radiolysis in airfree mixtures of 86 vol% ethanol and 14 vol% H_2O in neutral medium is briefly mentioned /19/. For illustration the observed transient absorption spectrum is presented in Figure 5.3.1. It shows a major absorption peak at 850 nm having two pronounced shoulders and a small maxima at < 250, 525 and 550 nm. The formation rate constant ($k = 4.3 \times 10^{9}$ $L.mol^{-1}.s^{-1}$) and the first order decay constant ($k_1 = 3.8 \times 10^{3}$ s^{-1}) were found to depend strongly on the viscosity of the solvent mixtures. The relatively long lived β-car$^{\bullet-}$ species were found to undergo mainly hydrolysis, forming stable final products.

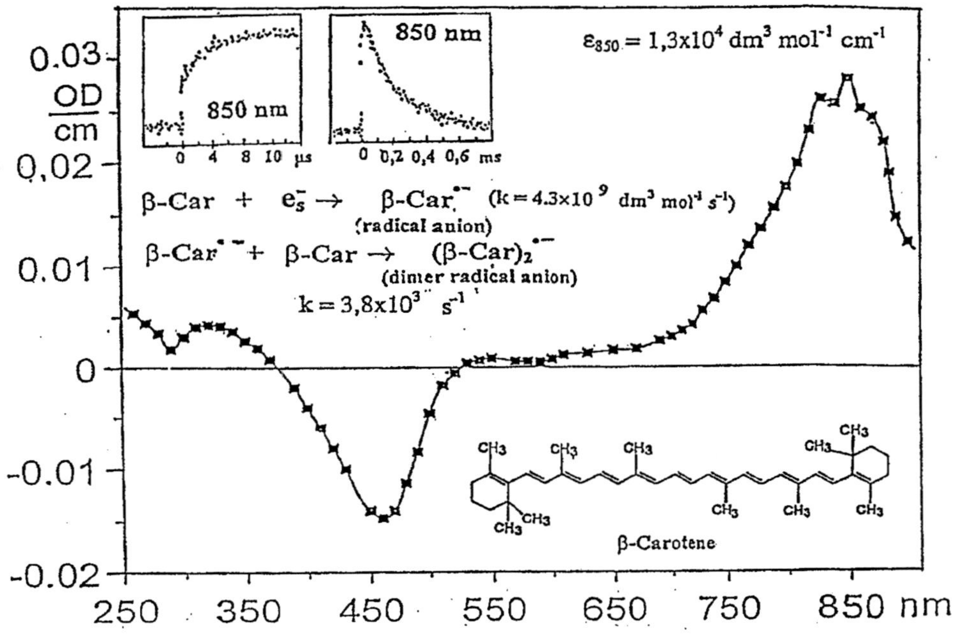

Figure 5.3.1. Absorption spectrum of β-car$^{\bullet-}$ radical anion resulting from airfree 5 x 10^{-5} mol/L β-carotene in a mixture of 86% ethanol and 14 % 4-times distilled water. OD/cm-values are normalized to 10 Gy. *Insert:* formation and decay kinetics and reactions. (Reprinted from Radiat.Phys.Chem.55, 395-398, 1999, by N.Getoff: Radical anion of β-carotene studied by pulse radiolysis in ethanol-water and tert-butanol-water mixtures, with permission from Elsevier).

Using DMSO as an appropriate solvent for β-car in aerated media, further pulse radiolysis experiments of β-carotene radical cation β-car$^{\bullet+}$ generation have been reported /20/. The absorption spectrum shows in the range about 550 nm the successively, strongly quenched triplet absorption spectrum of β-carotene (^{3}β-car) and simultaneously the time depending raising of the main absorption peak of β-car$^{\bullet+}$ at 942 nm (ε= 1.6x10^4 L.mol^{-1}.cm^{-1}) illustrated in Figure 5.3.2.

The major involved reactions are.

DMSO $\rightsquigarrow$ DMSO$^{\bullet+}$ + e_s^- + further species (5.14)

DMSO$^{\bullet+}$ = e_s^- = 1.3 (5.15)

$O_2 + e_s^- \rightarrow O_2^{\bullet-}$ (5.16)

DMSO$^{\bullet+}$ + β-car → DMSO + β-car$^{\bullet+}$ (k = 4.8 x 10^8 L.mol^{-1}.s^{-1}) (5.17)

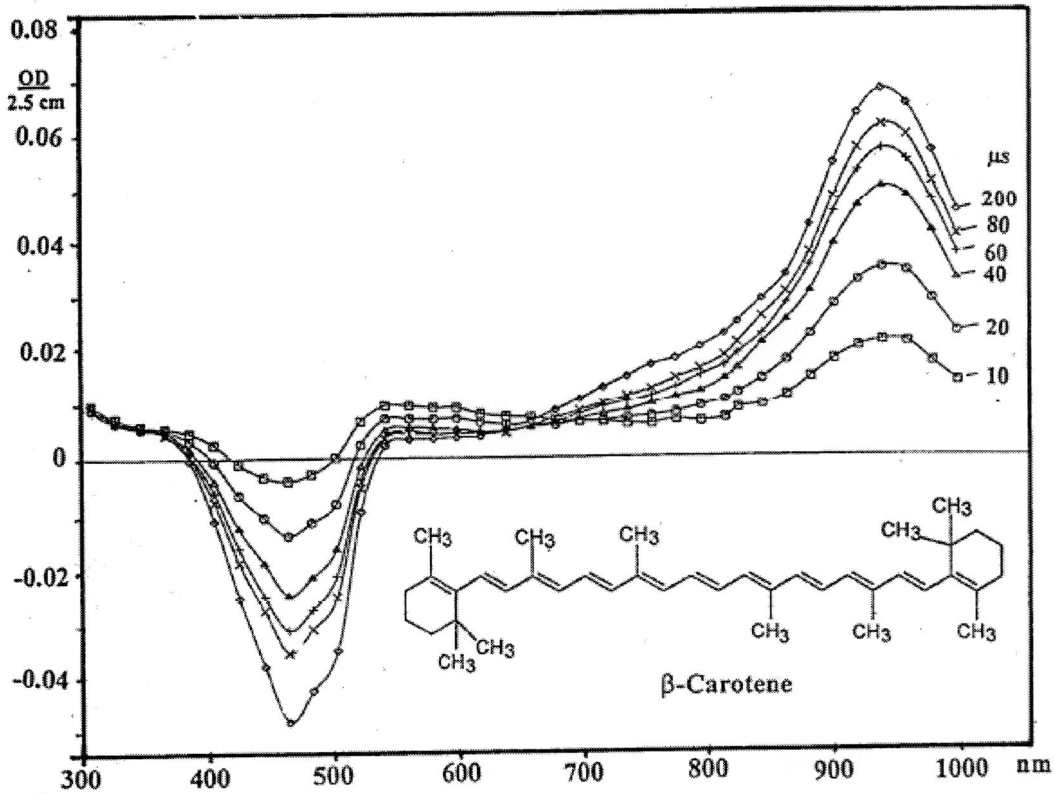

Figure 5.3.2. Transient absorption spectra of β-car$^{\bullet+}$ resulting from 1.5 x 10^{-5} mol/L β-carotene in DMSO in the presence of oxygen. (Reprinted from Radiat.Res.**154**, 692-696, 2000, by N.Getoff: Pulse radiolysis studies of β-carotene in oxygenated DMSO solution. Formation of β-carotene radical cation, with permission of Radiation Research Journal).

It was further established, that β-car$^{\bullet+}$ species disappear exclusively by first-order reaction ($k_1 = 2.1 \times 10^{3}\ s^{-1}$), probably by two processes: (1) at low substrate concentration by hydrolysis (this is important in biological point of view) and (2) at higher concentrations also by formation of a dimer radical cation (eq. 5.18):

$$DMSO^{\bullet+} + DMSO \rightarrow (DMSO)_2^{\bullet+} \qquad (5.18)$$

Under the applied experimental conditions the observed quenching process of ^{3}β-car by oxygen at 525 to 660 nm ($k = 7 \times 10^{4}\ s^{-1}$) is leading to the formation of singlet oxygen ($^1O_2$), which can also contribute to an additional formation of β-car$^{\bullet+}$ transients:

e.g. $$^1O_2 + \beta\text{-car} \rightarrow O_2^{\bullet-} + \beta\text{-car}^{\bullet+} \qquad (5.19)$$

Finally, it is noted, that the above mentioned transients generated from the vitamins C, E and β-carotene are certainly playing an essential role in human organism.

5.4. References

[1] Machlin L.J. (ed.) 1990, Handbook of Vitamins, Marcel Dekker, Inc. New York and Basel

[2] Bielski B.H.J., Comstock D.A. and Bowen R.A., 1991, Ascorbic acid free radicals. I. Pulse radiolysis study of optical absorption and kinetic properties, *J.Am.Chem.Soc.* 93, 5624-5628.

[3] Bielski B.H.J., 1982, Chemistry of ascorbic acid radicals, *Am.Chem.Soc., Adv.Chem.Ser.* 200, 81-100.

[4] Schöneshofer M., 1972, Pulse radiolysis studies of oxidation of ascorbic acid by OH radicals and halide radical anion complexes in aqueous solutions, Z.Naturforsch. 27b, 649-659.

[5] Schuler R.H., 1977, Oxidation of ascorbic anion by electron transfer to phenoxyl radicals, *Radiat.Res.* 69, 417-433.

[6] Cabelli D.E., Bielski B.H.J. and Seib B.A., 1984, A pulse radiolysis study of the oxidation of methyl substituted ascorbates, *Radiat.Phys.Chem.* 23, 419-429.

[7] Laroff G.B., Fessender R.W. and Schuler R.H., 1972, The electron spin resonance spectra of radical intermediates in the oxidation of ascorbic acid and related substances, *J.Am.Chem.Soc.* 94, 9062-9072.

[8] Getoff N., Platzer I. and Winkelbauer C., 1999, Transients and cooperative action of β-carotene, vitamin E and C in biological systems in vitro under irradiation, *Radiat.Phys.Chem.* 55, 699-704.

[9] Getoff N., 2001, Cytostatica efficiency enhancement by vitamins C, E and β-carotene under irradiation. State of the art., *Radiat.Phys.Chem.* 60, 351-358.

[10] Bisby R.H. and Parker A.W., 1991, Reaction of the α-tocopherol radical in micellar solutions studied by nanosecond laser flash photolysis, *FEBS* 290, 205-208.

[11] Cooper T.K. and Walker D.C., 1971, Free ion yield in the radiolysis of dimethylsulfoxide, *Canad.J.Chem.* 49, 2248-2253.

[12] Getoff N., Solar S., Richter U.B. and Haenel M.W., 2003, Pulse radiolysis of pyrene in apriotic polar organic solvents: simultaneous formation of pyrene radical cations and radical anions, *Radiat.Phys.Chem.* 66, 207-214.

[13] Getoff N., 2000, unpublished results.

[14] Dawe E.A. and Land E.J., 1975, Radical ions derived from photosynthetic polyens, *J.Chem.Soc., Faraday* Trans.I, 71, 2162-2169.

[15] Almgren M. and Thomas J.K., 1980, Interfacial electron transfer involving radical ions of carotene and diphenylhexatriene in micelles and vesicles, *Photochem. Photobiol.* 31, 329-335.

[16] Lafferty J., Roach C.A., Sinclair R.S. and Truscott T.G., 1977, Absorption spectra of radical ions of polyenes of biological interest, *J.Chem.Soc., Faraday Trans.*I, 416-419.

[17] Bensasson R.V., Land E.J. and Truscott T.G., 1983, Flash photolysis and pulse radiolysis. Contributions to the chemistry and biology and medicine, Pergamon Press, Oxford.

[18] Siehs H. and Strahl, W., 1995, Vitamins E,C and β-carotene and other carotenoids and antioxidants, *Am.J.Clin.Nutr.*(Suppl.), 1315-1321.

[19] Getoff, N., 1999, Radical anion of β-carotene studied by pulse radiolysis in ethanol-water and tert-butanol-water mixtures, *Radiat.Phys.Chem.*55, 395-398.

[20] Getoff, N., 2000, Pulse radiolysis studies of β-carotene in oxygenated DMSO solution, *Radiat.Res.*154, 692-696.

Chapter 6

Protection of Cell Membrane Damage by Antioxidant Vitamins

In general the cell membrane (thickness 7-10 nm) consist of proteins and lipids (20 – 25 %), vitamins (C, E, β-car, 2 – 5 %) in addition to carboxylic acids and water. The membrane structure is variable and depends on its origin and the specific function of the cell.

The degradation of the cell membrane by attack of oxidizing species (OH, $O_2^{\bullet -}$, $ROO^{\bullet}$ etc.) can be protected by a cascade electron transfer process between the antioxidant vitamins /1,2/. Based on the present knowledge the following pathway is involved: β-car contained in distinct areas at the outer layer of the cell membrane is getting first in contact with oxidizing agents (e.g. OH-radicals). The ejected electron from β-car neutralizes the OH-attack by forming the passive OH^- ion and a rather strong oxidizing β-$car^{\bullet +}$ (radical cation). The last one could destroy the membrane layer, because of its strong oxidizing properties, but it is regenerated to β-car by electron transfer from vitamin E (formation of vit.$E^{\bullet +}$). In turn each vit.$E^{\bullet +}$ (radical cation) is regenerated to vit.E by electron provided from vitamin C (ascorbate, AH^-). The resulting $AH^{\bullet}$ radicals undergo disproportion, resulting in DHA (dehydroascorbate). The protection of the cell membrane damage by a cascade electron transfer is visualized by scheme 6.1.

The rate constants of the involved electron transfer reaction were determined by pulse radiolysis in DMSO solutions and are also presented in the scheme 6.1.

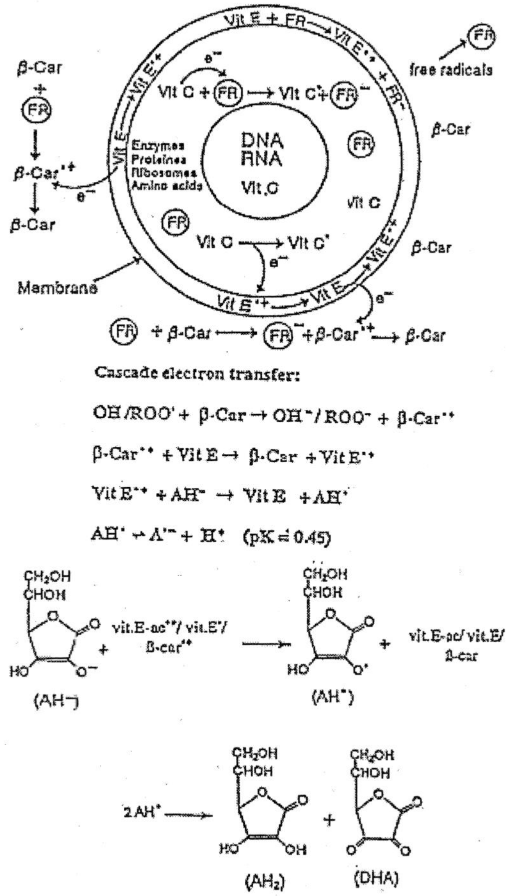

Reactions of the cascade electron transfer	k ($L.mol^{-1}.s^{-1}$)
$DMSO^{\bullet+}$ + β-Car. → DMSO + β-$Car^{\bullet+}$	2.3 x 10^9
β-$Car^{\bullet+}$ + Vit.E → β-Car. + $Vit.E^{\bullet+}$	2.7 x 10^9
$Vit.E^{\bullet+}$ + AH^- → Vit.E + $AH^\bullet$	3.1 x 10^9

Scheme 6.1. Cascade electron transfer from vitamin C → E → β-carotene and rate constants of the involved reactions. (Reprinted from Radiat.Phys.Chem.60, 351-358, 2001, by N.Getoff: Cytostatica efficiency enhancement by vitamins C, E and β-carotene under irradiation. State of the art, with permission from Elsevier).

6. References

[1] Getoff N., 2001, Cytostatica efficiency enhancement by vitamins C, E and β-carotene under irradiation. State of the art, *Radiat.Phys.Chem.* 60, 351-358.

[2] Getoff N., 2007, Anti-aging and aging factors in life. The role of free radicals, *Radiat.Phys.Chem.*76, 1577-1586.

Chapter 7

Synergistic Effect of Vitamin C, E And β-Carotene on Cytostatica and the Role of Oxygen

As already indicated, the oxidant vitamins, C, E and β-carotene act as electron donor. These processes are studied under the influence of ionizing radiation as a pathway for generation of free radicals. These ones can principally effect the activity of cytostatica by electron-transfer process under appropriate conditions.

It has been observed, that MMC-efficiency is strongly enhanced in the presence of the previously mentioned three vitamins by electron transfer process causing a synergistic effect /1/. The same synergistic action of the antioxidant vitamins on MMC was also observed on leukemia cells (HL 60) /2/ as well as on human lymphoblastic cell line /3/. Investigating the role of oxygen in combined systems, containing MMC and antioxidant vitamins, it was established, that the synergistic effect by the three vitamins in the presence of oxygen was under given conditions even much stronger expressed, than in airfree media. From the courses of the survival curves shown in Figure 7.1, the ΔD_{37}-values (Gy; see also insert Figure 7.1) are calculated in the absence and in the presence of air /1,4/. The negative ΔD_{37}-values (Gy) indicate the antitumor efficiency of the system. Similar results have been previously reportet /1,5/.

The presented data clearly demonstrate the role of oxygen on the MMC-antitumor effect in the presence of the three vitamins. This can be explained by the formation of the various oxidized forms of MMC and their biological action as already discussed in chapter 4.2.1. In addition to this also the peroxide formed in the presence of air can contribute to the observed effect.

As mentioned before (Chapter 4.2.) by means of pulse radiolysis studies in aqueous solutions (pH ~ 7.4), containing MMC and various oxygen concentrations, it was established, that with increasing O_2-content in the solution an electron-transfer from $MMC^{\bullet-}$ (semiquinone species) to O_2 takes place, resulting in the formation of peroxyl radicals ($O_2^{\bullet-}$) as shown in Figure 4.2.4.

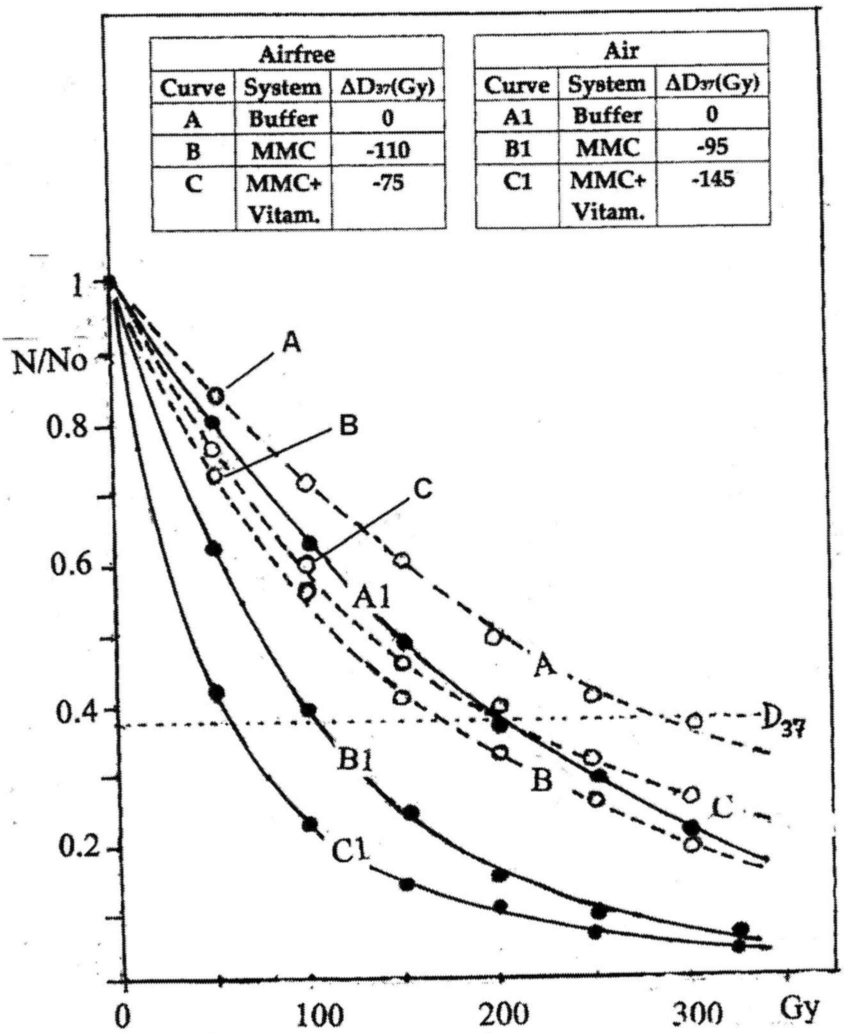

Figure 7.1. Survival curves (N/N0-ratio as a function of absorbed radiation dose (Gy) of Escherichia coli bacteria (AB 1157) at pH = 7.4. In airfree media, curves: A, B and C,as well as in the presence of air, curves: A1, B1 and C1; [MMC] = 2.5 x 10 -6 mol/L;[vitamins] = 1 x 10 -4 mol/L each of Vit.C, E and β-carotene. Insert: ΔD37-values of theindividual series. Applied dose rate: Dγ= 120 Gy/min

$$k(MMC^{\bullet -} + O_2 \rightarrow MMC + O_2^{\bullet -}) = 2 \times 10^9 \text{ L.mol}^{-1}.\text{s}^{-1} \quad (7.1)$$

The effect of vitamin C, E-acetate and β-carotene was also observed in sanazole (AK-2123) system in the frame of experiments in vitro (E.coli bacteria AB-1157) /6/. The antioxidant vitamins were applied with sanazole individually or in appropriate mixtures in airfree media (acting species: 44% e_{aq}^-, 10% H, 46% OH) as well as in media saturated with N_2O (90% OH, 10% H) or air (46% OH, 54% $O_2^{\bullet -}$). Under the given conditions the addition of vitamin C, as an efficient electron donor, led in all cases to a very strong increase of sanazole activity namely: in airfree media 2-fold, in presence of N_2O 1.5-fold and in the presence of air 2-fold. The effect of vitamin E-acetate and β-carotene as well as mixtures of them depends on the respective effect of the free radicals acting in the system. In airfree media the addition of vit.E-acetate or β-carotene causes a reduction of the sanazole activity.

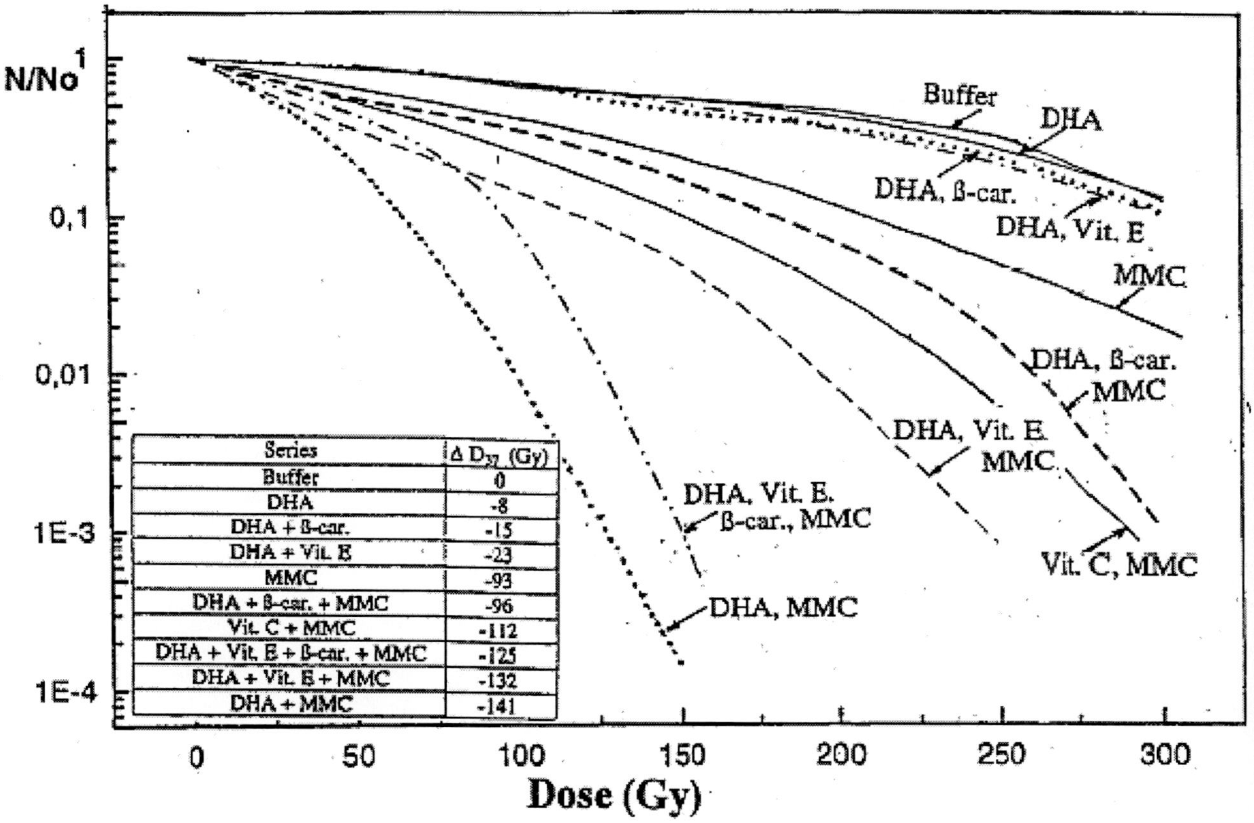

Series	Δ D_{37} (Gy)
Buffer	0
DHA	-8
DHA + ß-car.	-15
DHA + Vit. E	-23
MMC	-93
DHA + ß-car. + MMC	-96
Vit. C + MMC	-112
DHA + Vit. E + ß-car. + MMC	-125
DHA + Vit. E + MMC	-132
DHA + MMC	-141

Figure. 7.2. Synergistic effect of DHA and various mixtures of DHA with β-carotene, Vit.E and Vit.C on the MMC-efficiency in the presence of air at pH = 7.4, as a function of absorbed dose. Dose rate: 120 $Gy.min^{-1}$; [DHA] = [β-car] = [Vit.E] = 1 x 10^{-4} mol/L;[MMC] = 1 x 10^{-5} mol/L. Insert: ΔD_{37}(Gy)-values for the various mixtures.(Reprinted from In Vivo **18**, 795-798, 2004, by Kammerer C. and Getoff N., Synertistic effect ofdihydroascorbic acid in mixtures with vitamin E and β-carotene on mitomycin C under irradiation in vitro,with permission of the Journal).

The same effect was also observed in media saturated with N_2O. In aerated systems the addition of vit.E-acetate led only to a weak increase /6/.

The obtained results indicate a rather complicated reaction mechanism involved in the corresponding systems, where in the presence of air very likely the radical cations, $vit.E^{\bullet+}$ and $\beta\text{-car}^{\bullet+}$, play a role.

It is of interest to be mentioned, that from vitamin C generated dihydroascorbate (DHA), as presented in Figure 7.2 can likewise cause a strong synergistic action on MMC efficiency /7/. Figure 7.2. shows the individual synergistic behaviour of DHA on MMC as well as of DHA in mixtures with the vitamins C, E and β-carotene.

This effect is of interest in respect to the cancer treatment by implementation of MMC.

The exact mechanisms of the involved processes are not known, but are very likely based on electron transfer reactions.

7. References

[1] Getoff N., Platzer I. and Winkelbauer, C., 1999, Transients and cooperative action of β-carotene, vitamin E and C in biological systems in vitro under irradiation, *Radiat.Phys.Chem.*, 55, 699-704.

[2] Kammerer C., Czermak I., Getoff N. and Kodym R., 1999, Enhancement of MMC-efficiency by vitamin C, E-acetate and β-carotene under irradiation. A study in vitro, *Anticancer Res.*19, 5319-5322.

[3] Ortmann E.K., Mayerhofer T., Getoff N. and Kodym R., 2004, Effect of antioxidant vitamins in radiation-induced appoptosis in cells of human lymphoblastic cell line, *Radiat.Res.*161, 48-55.

[4] Getoff N., unpublished results.

[5] Getoff N., 2002, Effect of antioxidants and oxygen in radiotherapy; pp.99-105 in Progress of Radio-Oncology VII, Proceed. 7th Intern.Meeting on Progress of Radio-Oncology, Salzburg, Austria.

[6] Heinrich E. and Getoff N., 2000, Radiation-induced effect of vitamins C, E and β-carotene on sanazole efficiency. A study in vitro, *Anticancer Res.* 20, 3615-3618.

[7] Kammerer, C. and Getoff, N., 2004, Synergistic effect of dihydroascorbic acid in mixtures with vitamin E and β-carotene on mitomycin C under irradiation in vitro, in vivo 18, 795-798.

Chapter 8

Vitamins B-Series: General Remarks

The vitamins of the B-series show interesting biological properties under the influence of ionizing radiation. As mentioned before radiation is used to produce free radicals in aqueous solution, which are also generated in human organism. This makes possible to investigate their specific effect in biological systems. Having in mind the electronic structure of B-vitamins, one can assume, that practically all of them can eject electrons or/and transfer such to other systems, initiating e.g. redox-processes, causing synergistic effect on cytostatica etc. Some of them, like vitamin B1, B2, B3, etc. show also a strongly expressed antitumor ability. In order to understand better the manifold properties of this vitamin group and the effect of the acting free radicals in respect to their biological behaviour, in addition to the experiments in vitro, also chemical analysis of endproducts have been performed. In some cases the vitamin transients were also spectroscopically and kinetically characterized by pulse radiolysis technique. Based on all such data it is possible to get a deeper insight in the complicated biological processes and to indicate, that the resulting final products may also essentially contribute to observed biological sequences and side-effects.

8.1. Vitamin B1 (Thiamine)

Vitamine B1 (thiamine; 3-[4-amino-2-methyl-5-pyrimidinyl-methyl]-5-(hydroxylethyl)-4-methylthiazolinium chloride) is an essential nutrient, which is required for carbohydrate metabolism. In vitro it is converted into thiamine diphosphate, a coenzyme in the decarboxylation of α-keto acids.

Based on the molecular structure of vitamin B1 (vit.B1; see Figure 8.1.1.) and in accordance with previous experiences and knowledge /1/, it is expected that it should eject electron, when excited in singlet state. Some preliminary studies proved this assumption /2/.

Experiments in vitro (E.coli bacteria AB1157) demonstrated, that Vit.B1 in airfree media (acting species: 44% e_{aq}^-, 10% H, 46% OH) shows a rather strong antitumor ability, comparable to this of sanazole /3/. The mixture of both substrates, Vit.B1 and sanazole in airfree solution (series A, in Table 8.1.1.) did not lead to an increase of the ΔD_{37}-value. In aerated media, however, Vit.B1 acted as radiation protecting agent. This effect occur even in much stronger extent in solutions saturated with N_2O (conversion of e_{aq}^- into OH).

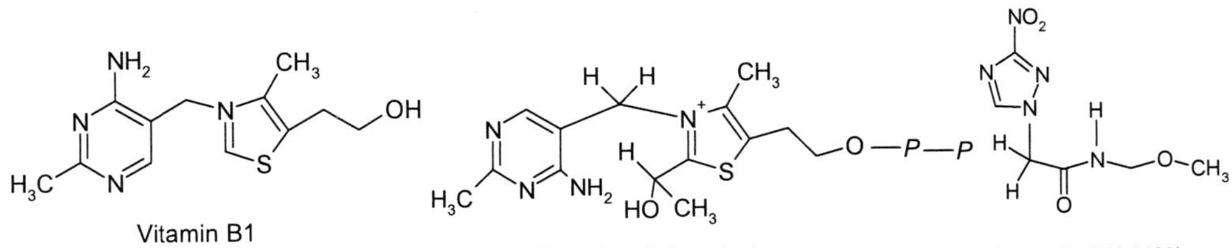

Vitamin B1 (Thiamine) — Thiamine diphosphate — Sanazole (AK-2123)

Figure 8.1.1. Formulas of vitamin B1, thiamine diphosphate and sanazole.

Under the same experimental conditions the mixture of Vit.B1 and sanazole showed a strong cytostatic effect (Table 8.1.1.)

Table 8.1.1. Series A: ΔD_{37}-values (Gy) of the systems: vitamin B1, sanazole and mixtures of both. Series B: ΔD_{37}-values (Gy) of sanazole as well as in mixtures of sanazole and antioxidant vitamins (C, E, β-carotene). The data of both series were obtained in different media

Series	System	ΔD_{37}-values (Gy)		
		Airfree 44% e_{aq}^-,10% H,46% OH	N_2O 10% H, 90% OH	Aerated 46% OH, 54% $O_2^{\bullet-}$
A	Buffer	0	0	0
	Vitamin B1	-151	+110	+14
	Sanazole	-123	-120	-46
	Sanazole+Vit.B1	-151	-149	-82
B	Sanazole	-55	-95	-75
	Sanazole+vit.C,E,β-car.	-140	-120	-50

The ΔD_{37}-values express the absorbed radiation dose (Gy), where the survival rate (N/N_0-ratio) of bacteria or cells used in the experiments, amounts to 37% after treatment. The negative values indicate the cytostatic ability of the system, whereas the positive ones show its radiation protection effect. N_0 means number of bacteria or cells before and N - after radiation treatment.

In aqueous mixtures (pH = 7.4) of sanazole and antioxidant vitamins, C, E and β-carotene (series B, Table 8.1.1.), quite different ΔD_{37}-values were reported for experiments in vitro (E.coli bacteria, AB 1157) although observed under similar experimental conditions but using a fresh bacteria strain /4/. Some data are presented in Table 7.1.1. for comparison. In all three media (airfree, N_2O, aerated) sanazole as well as the substrate mixtures in series B exhibit strong cytostatic properties, which are somewhat comparable with those of series A.

Similar investigations in vitro, concerning the effect of Vit.B1 and antioxidant vitamins (C, E, β-car.) on mitomycin C (MMC) under γ-ray treatment have been also reported /5/. Some data concerning the ΔD_{37}-values obtained by experiments in vitro (E.coli bacteia, AB 1157) in various aqueous media (pH 7.4) are presented in Table 8.1.2.

Table 8.1.2. ΔD_{37}-values (Gy) from experiments in vitro, showing the radiation induced effect of vit.B1 as well as by mixtures of vit.B1 and antioxidant vitamins (C, E, β-car.) on mitomycin C (MMC) in various aqueous media (pH = 7.4)

System	ΔD_{37}-vaues (Gy)		
	Airfree 44% e_{aq}^{-},10% H,46% OH	N_2O 10% H, 90% OH	Aerated 46% OH, 54% $O_2^{\bullet -}$
MMC	-72	-168	-34
MMC+vit.B1	-148	-80	-132
MMC+vit.B1+ vit.C,E,β-car.	-127	-217	-87

[MMC] = 1x10 $^{-6}$ mol/L; [vit.B1] = [vit.C] = [vit.E] = [β-car.] = 1x10 $^{-4}$ mol/L
dose rate: D_r=77 Gy/min; The reproducibility of the results depends on the concentration of used substrates, absorbed radiation dose and dose rate. These factors govern the concentration ratio between substrate and free radicals.

Obviously, the MMC efficiency is in airfree media highly increased in the presence of Vit.B1, but by the addition of antioxidant vitamins it is somewhat reduced, very likely due to interaction of the vitamins. On the contrary, in N_2O saturated media it is increased, but in the mixture MMC + Vit.B1 it is strongly reduced. However, by adding antioxidant vitamins the MMC-activity is increased. In solutions containing air, where only oxidizing radicals (OH and $O_2^{\bullet -}$) are operating the MMC-efficiency is about half reduced, however, in the presence of Vit.B1, it is 4-times enhanced. The addition of the vitamin mixture: B1 + antioxidant-vitamins led only to about 2.5-times increase.

Summing up, the presented results demonstrate, that vit.B1 exhibits in airfree media a rather strong cytostatic property. However, it does not influence the cytostatic effect of sanazole (Table 8.1.1). The mixture of vit.B1 and antioxidant vitamins contributes to an increase of the antitumor action of sanazole. In solutions saturated with N_2O vit.B1 acts as a potent radiation protecting agent, in contrast to the strong cytostatic ability of sanazole under the same conditions, where the vitamin-mixture (B1+C+E+β-car.) essentially contributes to the sanazole efficiency. In aerated media all observed ΔD_{37}-values show similar tendency as previously ones, but about 2-times reduced (see Table 8.1.1.).

Quite different influence of vit.B1 as well as of antioxidant vitamins (C, E, β-car.) on MMC is observed in the discussed three media (Table 8.1.2.). In airfree media MMC-efficiency is strongly increased in the presence of the vitamins. In N_2O-containing solutions vit.B1 reduces the MMC-action, but the mixtures of antioxidant vitamins causes an enhancement of the MMC-cytostatica action. In aerated media the addition of vit.B1 as well as that of the discussed vitamins is leading to a strong increase of MMC efficiency.

Based on these results it can be stressed, that vit.B1 as well as vit.B1 in mixture with antioxidant vitamins can essentially influence the cytostatic efficiency of sanazole and of MMC. This effect depends on several factors, such as the kind of the operating free radicals in a given process, but certainly also on the specific reactivity of the used cytostatica towards the individual free radicals, absorbed radiation dose (Gy) and dose rate (Gy/min) etc. There are still open questions concerning the reaction mechanism of the combined efforts: vitamins-cytostatica. The presented data are opening new pathways in this respect.

8.1. References

[1] Getoff, N., 1989, a review of the relationship between $Q(e_{aq}^-)$ and Q(F) of excited compounds in aqueous solution, Radiat.Phys.Chem.34, 711-719.

[2] Getoff, N., 2000, unpublished data.

[3] Heinrich, E. and Getoff, N., 2002, Influence of vitamin B1 on sanazole activity under irradiation. A strudy in vitro, Anticancer Res. 22, 927-930.

[4] Heinrich, E. and Getoff, N., 2003, Effect of vitamin B1 and mixtures of B1 with other vitamins on cytostatica efficiency of sanazole under irradiation. A study in vitro, Radiat.Phys.Chem. 67, 487-492.

[5] Heinrich, E. and Getoff, N., 2003, Mitomycin C activity effected by vitamins B1, C, E and β-carotene under irradiation with γ-rays, Z.Naturforsch. 58C, 244-248.

8.2. Vitamin B2 (Riboflavin)

Vitamin B2 (vit.B2; riboflavin, 7,8-dimethyl-10(1'-ribityl)-isoalloxazine) is content of various foods, such as meats, fish, seafood, milk, eggs, vegetables and fruits, but mostly in yeast. Vit.B2 is slightly soluble in water (~15 mg/100 ml), but the sodium salt of riboflavin-5'-phosphate (FMN) has high water solubility /1/. The formulas of riboflavin, FMN and FAD (flavin adenine dinucleotide) are shown in Figure 8.2.1. FMN and FAD are bioactive forms occurring in tissues and cells.

As previously established riboflavin (vit.B2) as well as other flavins are acting as electron donor by excitation in their singlet states /2,3/. Riboflavin in the coenzyme forms FMN and FAD can therefore operate as a mediator in the electron transfer in biological oxidation-reduction processes. The oxidases are soluble enzymes, which are content in the cell cytoplasm. Thereby NADP (nicotinamide-adenine-dinucleotide-phosphate) acts as initial electron acceptor, that mediates the electron to the flavoprotein, which transfers it directly to the molecular oxygen, forming peroxyl radical ($O_2^{\bullet-}$). The last one leads subsequently to peroxide formation.

$$O_2^{\bullet-} + O_2^{\bullet-} + 2H^+ \rightarrow H_2O_2 + O_2 \qquad (8.2.1.)$$

There are about 60 flavin containing enzymes, being flavoproteins, that follow the same biological pathway. Some of them contain FMN, but the most FAD as action group. From this very brief overview is obvious that vit.B2 plays an important role in various biological processes.

Further biological properties of vit.B2 have been established by specially designed experiments in vitro (model: E.coli bacteria AB 1157) /4/. In order to stimulate the action of free radical operating in human organism, the implemented systems were treated with γ-ray. The ΔD_{37}-values have been calculated from the corresponding survival curves, observed in various systems in oxygenated aqueous media (pH = 7.4) /4/. Under the applied experimental conditions oxydizing radicals only (46% OH and 54% $O_2^{\bullet-}$) are operating. It was established that in such environment vit.B2 acts as a very strong protecting agent towards the attack of

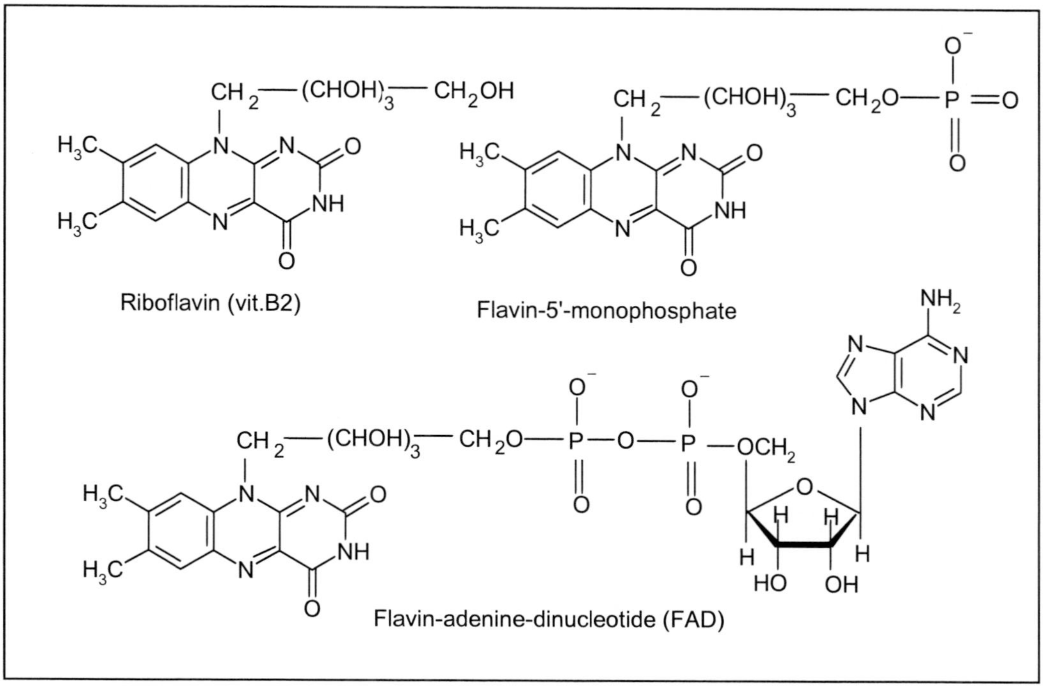

Figure 8.2.1. Formulas of vit.B2, FMN and FAD.

the oxidizing free radicals. This effect is even increased in the presence of ascorbate (vit.C).Interesting observation has been made, that under the influence of radiation in aerated media, vit.B2 completely suppresses the cytostatic activity of MMC. Further more, in the presence of both vitamins, vit.B2 and C, the cytostatic action of MMC is converted into a very efficient radiation protection effect. Some data illustrating this subject matter are presented in Table 8.2.1.

Table 8.2.1.: ΔD_{37}(Gy)-data concerning the effect of vit.B2 as well as of Vit.C, MMC and mixtures of them

System	Concentration (mol/L)	ΔD_{37}(Gy)
Buffer	(pH=7.4)	0
Vit.B2	10^{-5}	+ 40
Vit.C	10^{-4}	+ 60
MMC	3×10^{-7}	- 20
VitB2+MMC	as above	+ 15
Vit.B2+Vit.C+MMC	as above	+ 80

In the frame of preliminary experiments in vitro (E.coli bacteria AB 1157) in airfree media (pH = 7.4), where the operating radicals are: 44% e_{aq}^{-}, 10% H and 46% OH the presence of vit.B2 increases the cytostatic action of MMC /5/. This effect can be explained by an electron transfer from vit.B2 to MMC (generation of $MMC^{\bullet -}$ semiquinone), which is known as a very potent cytostatic transient (see chapter 4.2.).

The very efficient electron transfer from electron adducts of pyrimidine nucleotides to riboflavin (vit.B2), flavin adenine dinucleotid (FAD) and chloranil has been studied by pulse radiolysis /6/. The captured electron from pyrimidine electron adducts, induced in irradiated cell, would reduce a possible repair of the damaged target by inhibition of radical ion pair recombination. Riboflavin and FAD may act as radio-sensitizer in DNA damage process.

8.2. References

[1] Cooperman, J.M. and Lopez, R., 1990, pp283-310 in *Handbook of Vitamins, 2nd Edition*, Machlin L.J., editor, Publ.Marcel Dekker, Inc., New York and Basel.

[2] Getoff, N., 1989, A review of the relationship between $Q(e_{aq}^-)$ and Q(F) of excited compounds in aqueous solution, *Radiat.Pys.Chem.*34, 711-719.

[3] Getoff, N., Solar, S. and Mc.Cormick, D.B., 1978, Photoejection of electrons from Flavins in polar media, *Science* 201, 616-618.

[4] Fuga, L., Kragl, M. and Getoff, N., 2004, Vitamin B2 (Riboflavin) and mixtures of vitamin B2 and C effects MMC efficiency in aerated media under irradiation, *Anticancer Res.* 24, 4031-4034.

[5] Getoff, N., 2005, unpublished results.

[6] Lu, Ch-Y., Lin W.-Z., Wang W.-F., Han Z.-H., Zeng Z.-D. and Yao S.-D., 2000, Kinetic observation of rapid electron transfer between pyrimidine electron adducts and sensitizers of riboflavin, flavin adenine dinucleotid (FAD) and chloranil: a pulse radiolysis study, Radiat.*Phys.Chem.*59, 61-66.

8.3. Vitamin B3 (Nicotinamide)

Vitamin B3 (nicotinamide, niacinamide, pyridine-3-carboxamide), nicotinic acid and a number of its metabolites occur widely in the nature /1/. Nicotinamide (vit.B3) plays an important biological role in redox reactions of the coenzyme couple NAD^+ (nicotinamide-adenine-dinucleotide) – NADH (nicotinamide-adenine-dinucleotide-phosphate), which belongs to the group of pyridinnucleotides (see Figure 8.3.1).

The electron transferring (equivalent to hydrogen transferring) enzymes, e.g. of fermentation, glycolyse and many other processes, contain dinucleotide as acting group.

In order to get a deeper understanding of the reaction mechanism of vit.B3 also pulse radiolysis studies have been performed. The transient absorption spectra and rate constants for the reactions of OH and e_{aq}^- with aqueous pyridine /2/, as well as those of carboxy, carboamido and pyridyl derivatives of pyridine where reported /3/.

For nicotinamide (vit.B3) has been established:

$$k(e_{aq}^- + \text{vit.B3}) = 2.4 \times 10^{10}\ \text{L.mol}^{-1}\text{s}^{-1}\ (\text{pH} = 7.5)$$

$$k(\text{OH} + \text{vit.B3}) = 1.5 \times 10^{9}\ \text{L.mol}^{-1}\text{s}^{-1}\ (\text{pH} = 9)$$

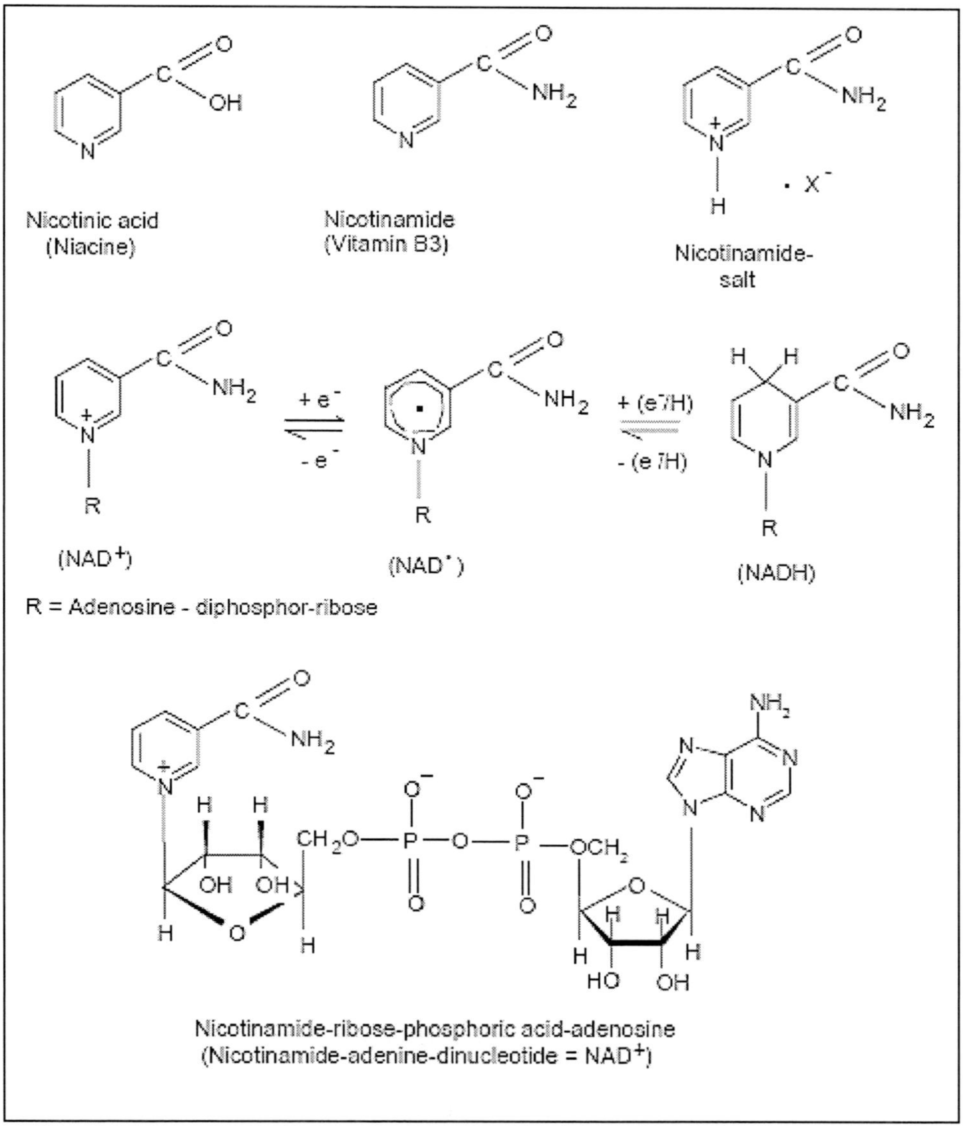

Figure 8.3.1. Formulas of nicotinic acid, vitamin B3, nicotinamide salt as well as redox-reactions of the coenzyme couples NAD^+/NADH.

The reactivity of OH, H and e_{aq}^- with nicotinic acid and nicotinamide and the resulting transients have also been reinvestigated, probable reaction mechanisms were proposed /4/.

The reversible two steps electron transfer (Figure 8.3.1, as well as eqs. 8.3.1 and 8.3.2) involving the couple NAD^+ - NADH has also been subject of pulse radioysis studies /5 and refs.therein/.

$$NAD^+ + e^- \leftrightarrow NAD^\bullet \qquad (8.3.1.)$$

$$NAD^\bullet + e^- + H^+ \leftrightarrow NADH \qquad (8.3.2.)$$

For the one electron oxidation of NADH by various phenoxyl radicals and phenothiazine radical cations rate constants in the range of 10^5 to 10^8 $L.mol^{-1}s^{-1}$ were found, depending on the redox potential of oxidizing species. Thereby, $NAD^{\bullet}$ transient is quantitatively formed, with no indication for the existence of its protonated form, $NADH^{+}$.

On the other hand one-electron reduction of $NAD^{\bullet}$ species to form NADH has not been observed under the applied experimental conditions.

In general, radiosensitizers for cancer cells are rather toxic, however, the toxicity of vit.B3 is very low. Otherwise it has been established, that vit.B3 disposes of well pronounced cytostatic properties /e.g. 6-9/. Based on these facts and in respect to the important biological role of vit.B3, discussed above, further experiments in vitro have been performed /10/.

Having in mind the action of antioxidant vitamins C, E and β-carotene as electron donor upon cytostatica (see chapter 7), the studies were focused on their synergistic action on the antitumor properties of vit.B3. The ΔD_{37}(Gy)-data of the experiments in vitro (E.coli bacteria, AB 1157) in aequeous media (pH = 7.4) under γ-ray irradiation are shown in Table 8.3.1.

In aerated media as already mentioned, H and e_{aq}^- are converted into peroxyl radicals. Hence, in such system are operating 46% OH and 54% $O_2^{\bullet-}$ species. It can be assumed, that the ejected electrons from antioxidant vitamins are also transformed into $O_2^{\bullet-}$ radicals. Therefore, the reported cytostatic increase in the mixture of vit.B3 and antioxidant vitamins can be attributed to oxidizing species.

Table 8.3.1.: Synergistic effect of vitamins: β-car., E and C on the cytostatic action of vit.B3 in oxygenated media (pH=7.4) under the influence of γ-irradiation. Escherichia coli bacteria (AB 1157) used as a model for experiments in vitro /10/.

System	D_{37}(Gy)	ΔD_{37}(Gy)
Buffer	160	0
NA	130	-30
β-car	215	55
NA + β-car	110	-50
vit.E	235	75
NA + vit.E	125	-65
vit.C	265	105
NA + vit.C	90	-70
NA + vits.C+E+β-car.	40	-120

[NA]=[β-car]=[vit.E]=[vit.C]= 1×10^{-4} mol/L.

Based on earlier results /11,12/ and considering the present knowledge, it is obvious, that the exact elucidation of the mechanisms of the interplaying reactions by free radicals in vitamin mixtures requires further investigations.

8.3. References

[1] van Eys, J., 1990, Nicotinic acid, pp.311-340 in Handbook of Vitamins by Machlin, L.J.(ed.), Marcel Dekker, Inc.New York.

[2] Cercek, B. and Ebert, M., 1967, Pulse radiolysis studies of the reaction of H and OH radicals and hydrated electrons with pyridine, Trans.Faraday Soc. 63, 1687-1698.

[3] Simic, M. and Ebert, M., 1971, Pulse radiolysis of aqueous solutions of carboxy, carbamido and pyridyl derivatives of pyridine, *Int.J.Radiat.Phys.Chem.* 3, 259-272.

[4] Solar, S., Solar, W., Getoff, N., Holcman, J. and Sehested, K., 1988, Reactivity of H, OH and e_{aq}^- with nicotinic acid. A pulse radiolysis study, *Radiat.Phys.Chem.* 32, 585-592.

[5] Grodkowsky J., Neta, P., Carlson, B.W. and Miller, L., 1983, One-electron transfer reactions of the couple NAD$^•$/NADH, *J.Phys.Chem.* 87, 3135-3138.

[6] Jonson, G.G., Kjellen, E., Pero, R.W. and Cameron, R., 1985, Radiosensitation effects of nicotinamide on malignat and normal mouse tissue, *Cancer Res.* 45, 3609-3614.

[7] Horseman, M.R., Brown, J.M., Hirst, V.K., Lemmon, M.J., Wood, P.J., Dunphy, E.P. and Overgaard, J., 1988, Mechanisms of action of the sensitive tumor radiosensitizer nicotinamide, Int.J.Radiat.*Oncol.Biol.Phys.* 15, 685-690.

[8] Horseman, M.R., Wood, P.J., Chaplin, D.J., Brown, .M. and Overgaard, J., , The potentation of radiation damage by nicotinamide in the SCCVII tumor in vivo, Radiat *Oncol.Biol.Phys.* 18, 49-57.

[9] Kjellen, E., Jviner, M.C., Collier, J.M., Johns, H. and Rojys, A., A therapoitic benefit from combinic normobaric carbogen or oxygen with nicotinamide in fractionated X-ray treatment, *Radiother.Oncol.* 22, 81-91.

[10] Getoff, N., 2003, Effect of vitamin C, E-acetate and β-carotene on the cytostatic activity of nicotinamide (vitamin B3), *In vivo* 17, 169-172.

[11] Steenken S., 1983, Purin bases, nucleosides and nucleotides: Aqueous solution redox chemistry and transformation reaction of their radical cations and e^- and OH-adducts, *Chem.Rev.*89, 503-520.

[12] Steenken S., 1992, Electron-transfer-induced acidity/basic and reactivity changes of purine and pyrimidine bases. Consequences of redox processes for DNA base pairs, *Free Radical Communs.*16, 349-379.

8.4. Vitamin B4 (Adenine)

Adenine (vitamin B4, vit.B4; 3,6-dihydro-6-aminopurine) plays a manifold biological role. It is a base, which upon creating a C-N bond with sugar (β-D-ribose) forms the nucleoside adenosine. In combination with phosphoric acid it results in adenosine-5-monophosphate (AMP) and appears as a component of DNA as well as of various co-enzymes. It has been observed, that by implementation of adenosine-5′-monophosphate (AMP) or adenosine-5′-triphosphate (ATP) the growth of tumors is inhibited /1,2/. The toxicity of 2-chlorodeoxy-adenosine, a nucleotide analogue, has been investigated in vitro (leukaemia cells) with respect to the therapy of patients with chronic lymphocitic leukemia /3/. On the other hand 2-fluoroadenine and a number of 6-methylpurine-nucleoside derivatives after some modification were tested in vitro (E.coli bacteria) in respect to their biological properties /4/.

As it has been already indicated, that compounds having certain functional groups (e.g. –NH_2, OH, $H_2PO_4^-$ etc.) are able to eject electrons from their excited state /5/. Hence, they can act as electron donor and can initiate biological redox-processes.

Special investigations were performed /6/, concerning the action of oxidizing (OH, $O_2^{\bullet-}$) and reducing free radicals (e_{aq}^-, H) in respect to the antitumor effect of vit.B4 and to its synergism to mitomycin C (MMC). As a model for the studies breast cancer cells (MCF-7) were implemented in various media at pH = 7.4. In aerated aqueous media (operating radicals: 46% OH, 54% $O_2^{\bullet-}$) using 2.5 µmol vit.B4 a highly pronounced radical protection effect was observed. However, the application of higher vitamin concentrations (50 µmol vit.B4) showed very strong cytostatic properties with regard to the cancer cells, as indicated in Figure 8.4.1, curve B. This effect as well as the synergistic influence of vit.B4 on the MMC activity is illustrated by the course of survival curves C, E and D, observed in aquous media in the presence of air (Figure 8.4.1).

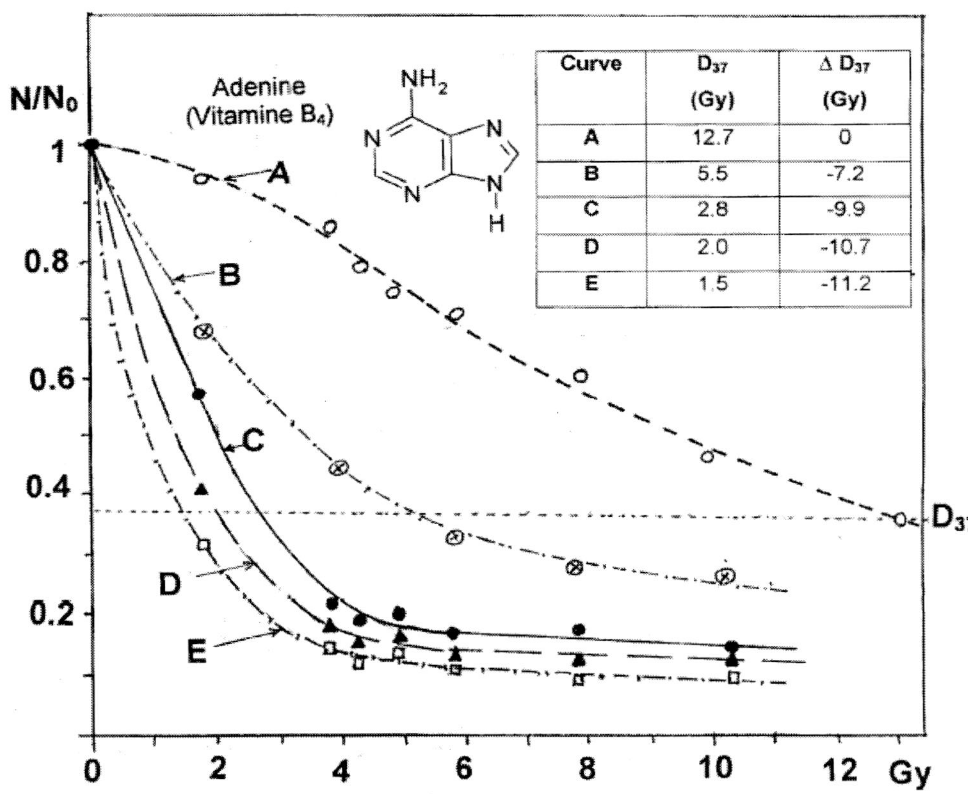

Figure 8.4.1. Survival curves (N/N0-ratio) as function of absorbed dose (Gy) for MCF-7 breast cancer cells in aerated media (2.5 x 10^{-4} mol/L O_2) at pH = 7.4. (A) Buffer, (B) 50 µmol vit.B4, (C) 5 µmol MMC, (D) 5 µmol MMC and 2 µmol vit.B4, (E) 5 µmol MMC and 50 µmol vit.B4.(Reprinted from Anticancer Res. 26, 3005-3010, 2006, by Hartmann, J. and Getoff, N., Radiationinduced effect of adenine (vitamin B4) on mitomycin C activity. In vitro experiments, with permission of the Journal).

Obviously, all ΔD_{37}-values (insert in Figure 8.4.1.) indicate that the involved components inhibit a strong antitumor property. The course of the survival curves (D) and (E) show the very essential synergisitic effect on MMC caused by 2 and 50 μmol vit.B4, respectively.

In media saturated with N_2O (acting species: 90% OH, 10% H) the added 2 and 50 μmol vit.B4 respectively, are likewise leading to an increase of MMC efficiency. In this case very likely the oxidized MMC transients, mentioned earlier, are involved.

Interesting data were reported by implementation of formate as a scavenger for OH and H radicals in anaerobic aqueous media (pH = 7.4). The resulting $^{\bullet}COO^-$ species can subsequently transfer electron to MMC, leading to a very strong increase of the $MMC^{\bullet-}$ yield and consequently to a very strong increase of the MMC efficiency /6/.

$$HCOO^- + OH \rightarrow {}^{\bullet}COO^- + H_2O \; (k = 2.7 \times 10^9 \; L.mol^{-1}.s^{-1}) \quad (8.4.1)$$

$$HCOO^- + H \rightarrow {}^{\bullet}COO^- + H_2 \; (k = 2.5 \times 10^8 \; L.mol^{-1}.s^{-1}) \quad (8.4.2)$$

$$MMC + {}^{\bullet}COO^- \rightarrow MMC^{\bullet-} + CO_2 \quad (8.4.3)$$

In this case also the radiation protection by vit.B4 was much stronger expressed and increased with the formate concentration.

It should be noticed that the reaction mechanisms caused by the oxidizing and reducing radicals are not yet completely understood. The complexity of the subject matter arises by the fact, that simultaneously with the above discussed effects, also a decomposition of vit.B4 takes place. Investigations in this respect showed that depending on the kind of acting free radicals different endproducts are formed /7/. The radiolysis of vit.B4 studied in aqueous solutions (pH = 7.4) saturated with argon (44% e_{aq}^-, 10% H, 46% OH) or with air (46% OH, 54% $O_2^{\bullet-}$) as well as with N_2O (90% OH, 10% H) resulted in decomposition yields, G(-vit.B4)-values, of 0.88, 1.16 and 1.45, respectively. As a main radiolytic product in all three media 8-hydroxyadenine (8-HOA) was determined. In aerated solutions in addition to 8-HOA also a mixture of aldehydes and carboxylic acids appeared to be main radiolytic products of vit.B4. The following set of reactions (Figure 8.4.2.) illustrates a probable mechanism for the vit.B4 radiolysis and product formation in the presence of air. Obviously, the final products depend on the position of the OH-attack on the vitamin molecule. It is interesting to note, that the highest 8-HOA yield has been observed in media saturated with N_2O, followed by those containing air. Based on the reactions in Figure.8.4.2. the formation of 8-HOA is initiated by OH-attack on vit.B4.

It has also been found that the radiation-induced degradation of 8-HOA in airfree media (44% e_{aq}^-, 10% H, 46% OH) is negligible. This fact refers to a possible involvement of regeneration reactions, as it has been earlier suggested for adenine radiolysis by Scholes et al. /8/. This process can be expressed by Figure 8.4.3.

As a conclusion can be stated, that vit.B4 can play at least a bifunctional role: (i) acting as a potent radical scavenger and (ii) showing an essential synergism towards MMC.

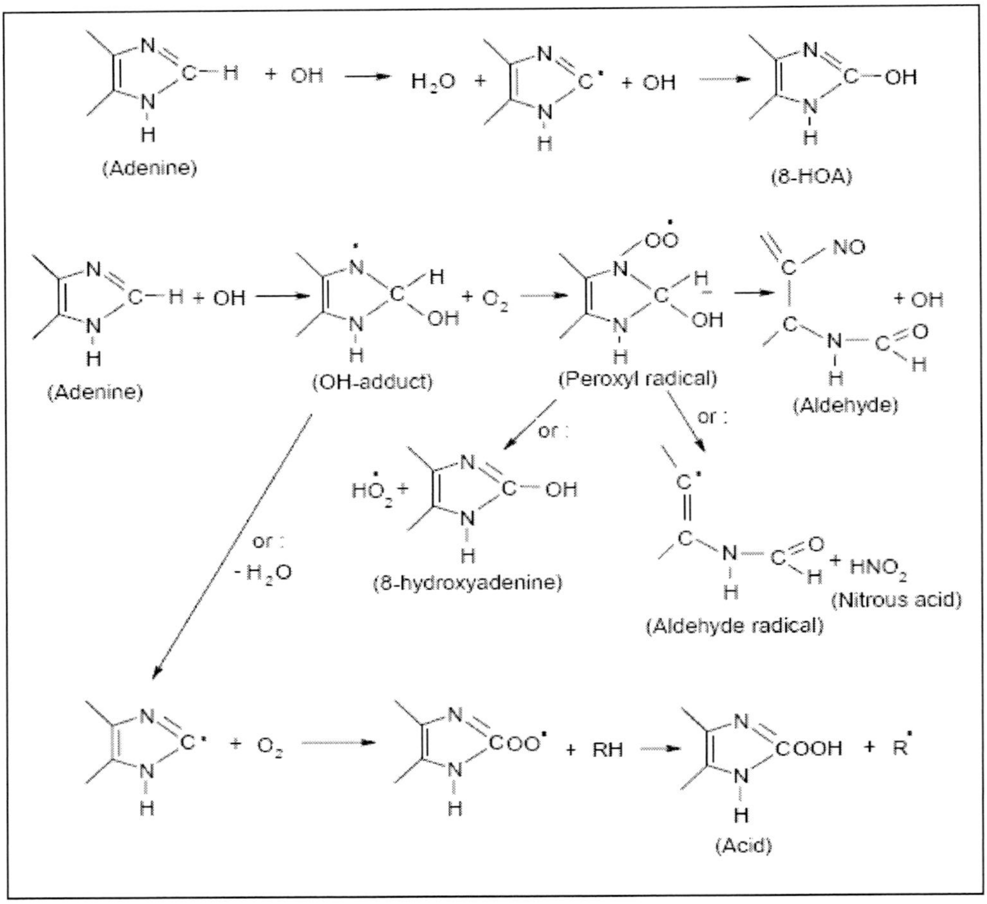

Figure 8.4.2. Probable reactions illustrating the formation of some radiolytic products of vit.B4 in aerated media. (Reprinted from Radiat.Phys.Chem. 76, 834-840. 2007 (Scheme 1), by Hartmann, J., Quint, R.M. and Getoff, N., 2007, Radiolysis of aqueous adenine (vitamin B4) and 8-hydroxyadenine, with permission of the Journal).

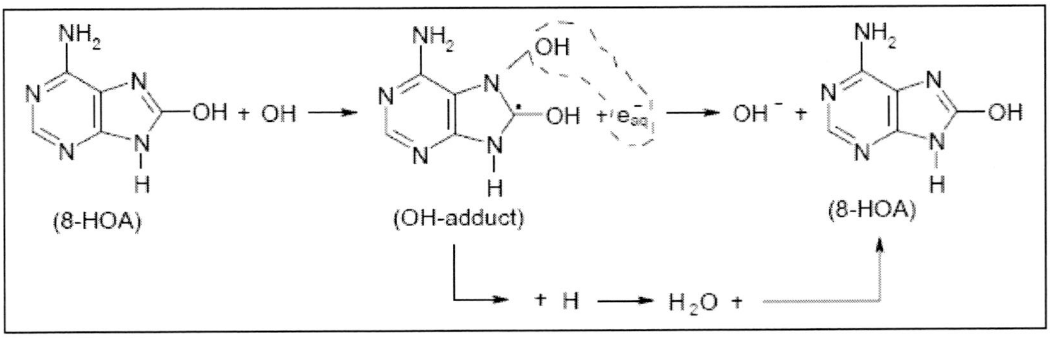

Figure 8.4.3. Degradation of 8-HOA (OH-attack) and regeneration of 8-HOA (reactions with eaq− and H-atoms). (Reprinted from Anticancer Res. 26, 3005-3010, 2006, by Hartmann, J. and Getoff, N., Radiation-induced effect of adenine (vitamin B4) on mitomycin C activity. In vitro experiments, with permission of the Journal).

8.4. References

[1] Rapaport, E. and Fontaine, J., 1989, Anticancer activities of adenine nucleotides in mice are mediated through expansion of erythrocyte ATP pools, *Proc.Nat.Sci.USA* 86, 1662-1666.

[2] Rapaport, E. and Fontaine, J., 1989, Generation of extracellular ATP in blood and its mediated inhibition of host weight loss in tumor-bearing mice, *Biochm.Pharmacol.* 38, 4261-4266.

[3] Lindemann, S., Lilienomark, J., Julinsson, G., Larsson, R. and Albertioni, F., 2004, Cytotoxicity and pharmakokinetics of cladribine metabolite, 2-chloroadenine in patients with leukaemia, *Cancer Lett.* 210, 171-177.

[4] Silamkoti, A.V., Allan, P.V., Hassan, E.E., Fowler, A.T., Sorscher, E.J., Parker, W.B. and Secrist, J.A., 2005, Synthesis of biological activity of 2-fluoroadenine and 6-methylpurinenucleoside analogues as prodrugs for suicide gene therapy of cancer, Nucleosides, Nucleotides, *Nucleic Acids* 24, 881-885.

[5] Getoff, N., 1989, A review of the relationship between $Q(e_{aq}^{-})$ and Q(F) of excited compounds in aqueous solution, *Radiat.Phys.Chem.* 34, 711-719.

[6] Hartmann, J. and Getoff, N., 2006, Radiation-induced effect of adenine (vitamin B4) on mitomycin C activity. In vitro experiments, *Anticancer Res.* 26, 3005-3010.

[7] Hartmann, J., Quint, R.M. and Getoff, N., 2007, Radiolysis of aqueous adenine (vitamin B4) and 8-hydroxyadenine, *Radiat.Phys.Chem.* 76, 834-840.

[8] Scholes G., Ward, J.F. and Weiss, J., 1960, Mechansim of the radiation-induced degradation of nucleic acid, *J.Molec.Biol.* 2, 379-391.

8.5. Vitamin B5 (Pantothenic Acid)

Vitamin B5 (vit.B5; 2,4-dihydroxy-3,3-dimethylbutyryl)-β-alanine) is an essential vitamin for the biosynthesis of coenzyme A in mammalian cells. It occurs ubiquitously in all animal and plant tissues. The richest common source is liver, but jelly of the queen bee contains 6 times as much as liver. Vit.B5 is a unstable, very hygroscopic viscous oil, freely soluble in water.

A number of papers are reporting about the many-sided biological properties of vit.B5 and its derivatives. Experiments in vitro as well as in vivo have shown that it exhibits an antioxidative effect (/1-3/) as well as protective properties against ionizing radiation (/4-6/). Additionally, vit.B5 protects or delays jurkat cells against UV-light apoptosis /7/. Further, having in mind the molecular structure of vit.B5 (see Figure 8.5.1.) and based on some preliminary experiments by the author, it can be expected that it is able to eject electrons from its singlet ecxited state /8,9/. Such property has been previously observed at antioxidant vitamins (C, E, β-carotene) and by their combination with cytostatica, e.g. MMC /10/.

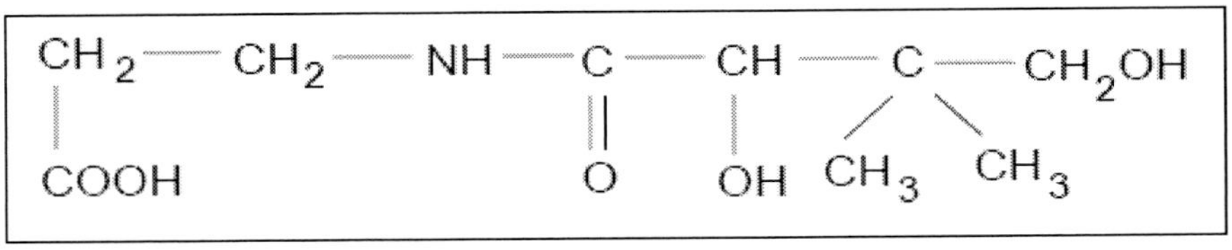

Figure 8.5.1. Formula of vitamin B5 (panthotenic acid)

Investigations concerning especially the antitumor properties of vit.B5 and its synergistic effect on MMC were performed under various conditions /9/. As a model for the experiments in vitro Escherichia coli bacteria (AB 1157) were used. The aim of the studies was focussed on the action of oxidizing (OH, $O_2^{\bullet-}$) and reducing free radicals (e_{aq}^-, H) on vit.B5 and MMC individually as well as on mixture of both. The free radicals were generated by implementation of γ-ray in appropriate media.

In Table 8.5.1. some data are shown of D_{37}-values, derived from the corresponding survival curves, observed in the mentioned systems /9/.

The results in Table 8.5.1. clearly demonstrate the strong expressed antitumor property (-ΔD_{37} values) of vit.B5, shown in series B, in comparison to those of MMC (series C) initiated by oxidizing free radicals (OH and $O_2^{\bullet-}$). In addition to this the synergism of vit.B5 on MMC (series D) appears to be also very strong.

In aqueous media saturated with argon (acting species: 44% e_{aq}^-,10% H,46% OH) the ΔOD-values were also reported /9/. In this case MMC-semiquinone ($MMC^{\bullet-}$) and MMC.OH (OH-adduct) are formed at about equal concentration, but a certain part of OH and e_{aq}^- are reacting with each other. In Table 8.5.2. some results in this respect are presented.

Table 8.5.1.: D_{37}- and ΔD_{37}-values derived from survival curves expressing the N/N_0-ratio as function of absorbed radiation dose (Gy), registered in aqueous media saturated with air or N_2O, respectively (pH=7.4). N_0 = number of bacteria before and N = number of bacteria after irradiation treatment. Series (A) buffer, series (B) $1x10^{-4}$ mol/L vit.B5, (C) $5x10^{-6}$ mol/L MMC and (D) mixture of both. Dose rate of γ-ray: 45 Gy/min /9/

Experimental series	1		2	
	Aerated media 46% OH, 54% $O_2^{\bullet-}$		Media saturated with N_2O 10% H, 90% OH	
	D_{37} (Gy)	ΔD_{37} (Gy)	D_{37} (Gy)	ΔD_{37} (Gy)
A	230	0	220	0
B	170	-60	175	-45
C	120	-110	105	-115
D	80	-150	55	-165

Table 8.5.2. N/N_0-values determined at 100 and 300 Gy absorbed radiation dose in aqueous media (pH=7.4) saturated with argon. Systems: (A) buffer, (B) $5x10^{-5}$ mol/L vit.B5, (C) $3x10^{-7}$ mol/L MMC and (D) mixture of both. Dose rate: 45 Gy/min. N_0 = number of E.coli bacteria before and N = number of bacteria after irradiation treatment

Series	N/N_0-values at:	
	100 Gy	300 Gy
A	0.97	0.63
B	0.81	0.46
C	0.90	0.55
D	0.76	0.34

(Remark: The lower is the N/N0-ratio, the higher is the antitumor efficiency compared to series A).

Table 8.5.3. G(-vit.B5)*) values obtained for degradation of 10^{-3} mol/L vit.B5 by various types of free radicals /11/

Free radicals	Acting radicals in %		
	Airfree media	Media saturated with N_2O	Aerated media
e_{aq}^-	44	---	---
H	10	10	---
OH	46	90	46
$O_2^{\bullet-}$	---	---	54
G(-vit.B5)	0.72	3.22	1.44

*) G-value = number of decomposed molecules per 100 eV absorbed energy.

The observed MMC-efficiency (series C) is somewhat lower (higher N/N_0-values) as this of vit.B5 (series B). However, the mixture of both shows the highest antitumor effect, indicating the synergism of vit.B5 to MMC.

Comparing the results presented in both Tables, it can be stressed, that in all investigated media the applied mixtures of vit.B5 and MMC show the highest antitumor efficiency compaired to their individual ability. Besides, this effect is in aerated media about double larger than in the other media, indicating the role of oxidizing transients in the present systems.

Nevertheless, the final products formed under the above experimental conditions are certainly involved in the observed biological effects. Their formation, resulting from the free radical attack on vit.B5, is briefly mentioned. The vit.B5 degradation under various conditions is illustrated by the data presented in Table 8.5.3.

The data in the above table indicate that the OH-radicals are the most powerful oxidation species, resulting in G(-vit.B5) = 3.22, followed by $O_2^{\bullet-}$, which is a rather slowly reacting species. In the airfree media about equal concentrations of reducing (e_{aq}^-, H) and oxidizing radicals (OH) are implemented in the process, the lowest degradation yield was observed. Thereby, the reactivity of both types of free radicals with each other competes with their attack on substrate.

As final products a mixture of aldehydes was established with the highest yield in aerated media, whereas in media saturated with N_2O or argon, the aldehyde yields were about one order of magnitude lower /11/. A mixture of carboxylic acids as well as ammonia were also found. In addition to this the formation of a not yet identified major product has been determined. Based on this observation it can be stated, that not only vit.B5 is playing a versatile role, but it seems that the products originating from its degradation very likely are involved in various biological processes.

The reaction mechanisms involved in the discussed system is rather complicated and is not yet understood. Obviously, several competition processes are involved, depending on the type of free radicals produced in a given media. Electron transfer from vit.B5 to MMC seems to play thereby an essential role.

For illustration of the complexity of the involved processes, some very probable primary reactions are presented in Figure 8.5.2.

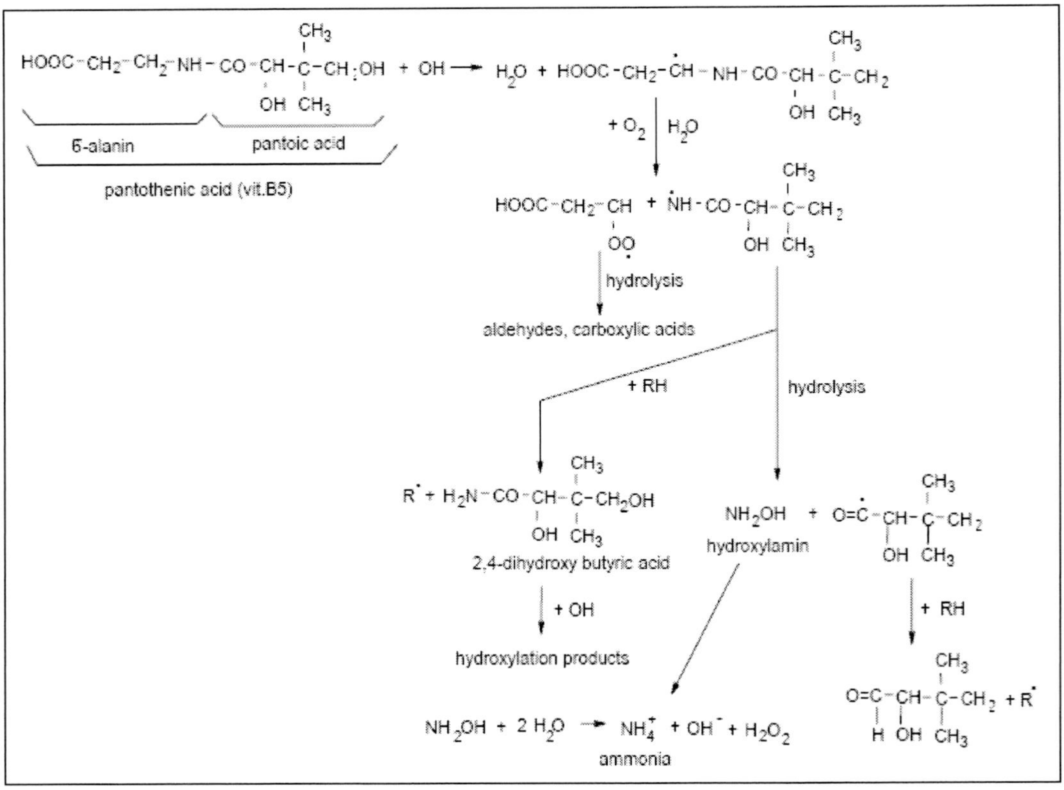

Figure 8.5.2. A selection of probable primary reactions of vit.B5 in aqueous, aerated media /11/.

Based on the observed final degradation products of vit.B5, the first reaction step is definitely initiated by OH radicals on several positions of the substrate molecule. The resulting vitamin transients are scavenged by oxygen, forming unstable peroxyl radicals, most of which undergo hydrolysis. As a final result of these processes several final products are formed, which are involved in biological processes.

8.5. References

[1] Yoshikawa, T., Furukawa, Y., Tamai, M., Murakawa, M. and Kondo, M., 1982, The increase of lipid peroxidation in experimental hepatitis in rats by carbon tetrachloride or D-galactosamine and its inhibition by pantethine, *J.Appl.Biochem.* 4, 228-233.

[2] Utno, L.J., 1991, Effect of pantethine on metabolism in myocardial mitochondria under conditions of deep hypothermia, *Bull.Exp.Biol.Med.* 111, 577-578.

[3] Slyshenkov, V.S., Moiseenokl, A.G. and Wojtczak, L., 1996, Noxious effects of oxygen reactive species on energy coupling process in Ehrlich ascites tumor mitochondria and the protection by pantothenic acid, *Free Radic.Biol.Med.* 20, 793-800.

[4] Artom, C., 1954, Effects of pantothenic acid and its analogs in radiation injury by P^{32}, *Proc.Soc.Exp.Biol.Med.* 86, 162-165.

[5] Szóràdy, I., Tóth, G. and Gazdag, I., 1965, X-ray protection by means of pantothenic acid, *Progr.Biochem.Pharmacol.* 1, 533-536.

[6] Slyshenkov, V.S, Omelianchik, S.N., Moiseenok, A.G., Pethusok, N.E. and Wojtczak, L., 1999, Protection by pantethenol and β-carotene against liver damage produced by low-dose γ-radiation, *Acta Biochim.Polon.* 46, 239-248.

[7] Slyshenkov, V.S., Pivocka, K., Sikora, E. and Wojtczak, L., 2001, Pantothenic acid protects jurkat cells against uv-light apoptosis, *Free Radic.Biol.Med.* 30, 1303-1310.

[8] Getoff, N., 1989, A review of the relationship between $Q(e_{aq}^-)$ and Q(F) of excited compounds in aqueous solution, *Radiat .Phys.Chem.* 34, 711-719.

[9] Schittl, H. and Getoff, N., 2007, Radiation-induced antitumor properties of vitamin B5 (pantothenic acid) and its effect on mitomycin C activity. Experiments in vitro, *Oncology Res.* 16, 389-394.

[10] Getoff, N., 2001, Cytostatica efficiency enhancement by vitamin C, E and β-carotene under irradiation. State of the art, *Radiat.Phys Chem.* 60, 351-358.

[11] Schittl, H., Quint, R.M. and Getoff, N., 2007, Products of aqueous vitamin B5 (pantothenic acid) formed by free radical reactions, *Radiat.Phys.Chem.* 76, 1594-1599.

8.6. Vitamin B6 (Pyridoxine Hydrochloride)

Vitamin B6 (vit.B6; pyridoxine hydrochloride; 5-hydroxy-6-methyl-3,4-pyridinedim-ethanol hydrochloride) is content in yeast, liver, cereals and in many foodstuffs. It is one of the components of the B6 complex. In the organism vit.B6 is transformed into pyridoxal and pyridoxamine, which are derivatives of the cofactor pyridoxal-5′-phosphate, required for numerous enzymatic reactions, mainly in amino acid metabolism (Figure 8.6.1.). The 5′-phosphorylated derivatives of pyridoxine, pyridoxal and pyridoxamine are dietary sources of vitamin B6 /1/.

The deficiency of vit.B6 is associated with an increased risk of cardiovascular disease, stroke and certain types of cancer (e.g. /2/ to /6/).

The reactivity of vit.B6 with OH-radicals is rather high. The reaction rate constants at pH = 3.6, k(OH + vit.B6) = 4.3×10^{9} $L.mol^{-1}s^{-1}$ and at pH = 7.2, k(OH + vit.B6) = 6.3×10^{9} $L.mol^{-1}s^{-1}$ were determined by pulse radiolysis method /7/.

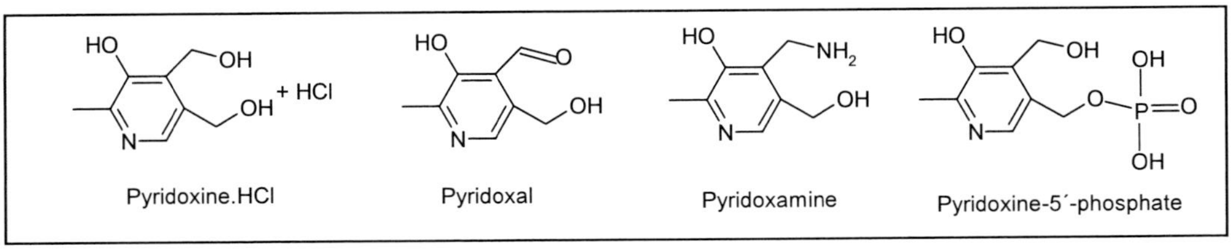

Figure 8.6.1. Formulas of pyridoxine, pyridoxal, pyridoxamine and pyridoxal-5´-phosphate.

Similar rate constants for the reaction of OH radicals with vit.B6 have been reported by other authors /8/. Somewhat higher values for the reactivity of e_{aq}^- with pyridoxine, $k = 2.2 \times 10^{10}$ $L.mol^{-1}s^{-1}$ at pH = 6.8 /7/ and for pyridoxal-5´-phosphate $k = 1.6 \times 10^{10}$ $L.mol^{-1}s^{-1}$ at pH ~ 7 /7/ have been found.

Table 8.6.1.: D_{37}- and ΔD_{37}-values derived from survival curves in vitro experiments (E.coli bacteria AB1157) performed in various aqueous media (pH ~ 7.4), containing vit.B6 individually and in mixtures with MMC and vit.C. (Dose rate: 100 Gy/min).

System	Airfree 44% e_{aq}^-,10% H,46% OH		Saturated with N_2O 10% H, 90% OH		Aerated 46% OH, 54% $O_2^{\bullet-}$	
	D_{37} (Gy)	ΔD_{37}(Gy)	D_{37} (Gy)	ΔD_{37}(Gy)	D_{37} (Gy)	ΔD_{37}(Gy)
Buffer	220	0	150	0	189	0
Vit.B6	125	-95	60	-90	164	-25
MMC	60	-160	25	-125	144	-45
MMC, Vit.B6	20	-200	260	110	99	-90
MMC, Vit.B6,Vit.C	165	-55	240	90	49	-140

Substrate concentration: [vit.B6] = 1×10^{-5} mol/L ; [MMC] = 5×10^{-6} mol/L ; [vit.C] = 1×10^{-5} mol/L.

In the frame of the studies, concerning the synergism of vitamins on cytostatic drugs, also experiments in vitro (E.coli bacteria AB 1157 used as a model) implementing vit.B6 and MMC (representative for cytostatica) have been performed /9/. The studies in aqueous airfree media are related to the fact, that cancer tissue contains only traces amounts of oxygen. Experiments were also performed in solutions saturated with N_2O (conversion of e_{aq}^- into OH) as well as in aerated media (transforming e_{aq}^- and H into peroxyl radicals, $O_2^{\bullet-}$), where different types of radicals are operative. It was established that vit.B6 exhibits, similar to MMC, in all media a strong pronounced antitumor effect (- ΔD_{37}-values). The ratio of the MMC-efficiency (ΔD_{37}-value) and that of vit.B6 in the above mentioned three different media is found to be: 1.7, 1.4 and 1.8, respectively. The data are presented in Table 8.6.1.

The mixture of vit.B6 and MMC in airfree solution showed the highest antitumor increase, indicating an synergistic effect of vit.B6 to MMC. But the addition of vit.C to the mixture of MMC + vit.B6 caused a strong efficiency reduction. This effect cannot be explained straight forward, since on one side vit.C acts as an efficient elelctron donor (favourizing $MMC^{\bullet-}$ formation), but on the other side MMC and OH species (having about the same concentration and rate constants) compete for e_{aq}^-. Based on this fact leads to less $MMC^{\bullet-}$ is formed. It is also conceivable, that the MMC-vit.B6-vit.C system is forming a kind of complex, which can also consume electrons. Further, special designed experiments are needed for elucidation of the interlaced reactions.

The synergistic effect can be likely explained by an electron transfer from vit.B6 to MMC (probably existing as a complex), resulting to the very active semiquinone, $MMC^{\bullet -}$. These species, as well known, can finally intercalate in the DNA of cancer cells, hindering their proliferation. On the other hand as mentioned before (Chapter 4), the OH adducts and peroxylradicals of MMC exhibit cytostatic properties likewise.

In aqueous media saturated with N_2O the system MMC-vit.B6 as well as MMC-vit.B6-vit.C show a strong radiation protecting effect, $\Delta D_{37} = 110$ and 90, respectively. On the other hand vit.B6 as well as MMC exhibit individually an essential antitumor property: -90 and -125, respectively (Table 8.6.1.). The involved reaction mechanism is rather complicated and presently not clear.

In aerated media all systems show cytostatic behaviour, but reduced by a factor of about 3.6 for the first three systems in comparison with the data in airfree solution. On the other hand the mixture of MMC-vit.B6-vit.C exhibit about 2.5-times higher cytostatic property for the same comparison.

Summing up, it can be stated, that vit.B6 has pronounced cytostatic properties, which are higher expressed in airfree media and are reduced by a factor of about 4 in aerated solutions. In addition to this, vit.B6 exerts a synergistic effect to MMC, increasing essentially its efficiency in the absence as well as in the presence of air and in media containing N_2O. Unexpectedly the MMC-vit.B6 as well as MMC-vit.B6-vit.C-system in solution saturated with N_2O, act as a perfect radiation protecting agent (ΔD_{37} = +110 and + 90, respectively; Table 8.6.1.).

It is obvious, that the radicals: e_{aq}^-, H, OH, $O_2^{\bullet -}$ play a crucial role in all discussed systems. The reaction mechanisms are rather complicated and are not clear yet. In addition to this it should be mentioned, that the radiolytic products, originating from the corresponding systems, are certainly involved in the observed processes and are effecting the observed results.

8.6. References

[1] Said, H.M. and Mohammed, Z.M., 2006, Intestinal absorption of water soluble vitamins: an update. *Curr.Opin.Gastroenterol* 22, 140-146.

[2] Setiwan, B., Giraud, D.W. and Driskell, J.A., 2000, Vitamin B6 inadequacy is prevalent in rural and urban Indonesian children. *J.Nutr.* 130, 553-558.

[3] Robinson, K., Arheart, K., Refsum, H., Brattström, L., Boers, G., Ueland, P., Ribba, P., Palma-Reis, R., Meleady, R., Daly, L., Witteman, J. and Graham C., 1998, Low circulating folate and vitamin B6 concentrations: risk factors for stroke, peripheral vascular disease and coronary artery disease. *Circulation* 97, 437-443.

[4] Ronnenberg, A.G., Goldman, M.B., Aitken, I.W. and Xu, X, 2000, Anemia and deficiencies of folate and vitamin B6 are common an vary with season in Chinese woman of childbearing age, *J.Nutr.* 130, 2703-2710.

[5] Lin, P.T., Cheng, C.H., Liaw, Y.P., Lee, B.T., Lee, T.W. and Huang, Y.C., 2006, Low pyridoxal-5′-phosphate is associated with increased risk of coronary artery disease, *Nutrition* 22, 1146-1151.

[6] Ames, B.N., 1999, Cancer prevention and diet: help from single nucleotide polymorphisms, *Proc.Natl.Acad.Sci.USA* 96, 12216-12218.

[7] Moorthy, P.N. and Hayon, E., 1975, One electron redox reactions of water soluble vitamins, III. Pyridoxine and pyridoxal phosphate (vitamin B6), *J.Am.Chem.Soc.* 97, 2048-2051.

[8] Greenstock, C.L. and Shierman, E., 1975, Radiosensitivity and hydroxyl radical reactivity of phosphate esters as measured by radiation-induced dephosphorylation, *Int.J.Radiat.Biol.Relat.Stud.Phys.Chem.Med.* 28, 1-11.

[9] /9/ Svoboda, B. and Getoff, N., 2002, Vitamin B6 and C and mitomycin C-efficiency under irradiation, *Anticancer Res.* 22, 949-952.

8.7. Vitamin B11 (Folic Acid)

Folic acid (vitamin B11, vit.B11; N-[4-[[2-Amino-1,4-dihydro-4-oxo-6-pteridinyl]methyl]benzoyl]-L-glutamic-acid) is a liver lactobacillus casei factor, hematopoietic vitamin, which is present, free or in combination with one or more molecules of L(+)-glutamic acid in liver, kidney, mushrooms, spinach, yeast, green leaves, grasses etc. /1/. It is slightly soluble in cold water (1.6 mg/L at 25°C), but is better soluble in aqueous alkaline or bicarbonate media and is composed of 6-methylpterin, 4-aminobenzoic acid and glutamic acid (Figure 8.7.1.).

Folate is a generic term for cofactor 5,6,7,8-tetrahydrofolate (THF; Figure8.7.1.), which is involved in the biosynthesis of purines, thymidylate, pantothenate, methionine etc. Folate deficiency has been linked to birth defects, cancer, cardiovascular disease and other illnesses (see e.g. /2/).

In addition to THF also 7,8-dihydrofolate is playing a versatile role, e.g. 7,8-dihydrofolate reductases in soybean /3/, carrot /4/, sunflower /5,6/ etc. It has been established that the plants contain the bifunctional dihydrofolate-reductase-thymidylate synthase /6/.

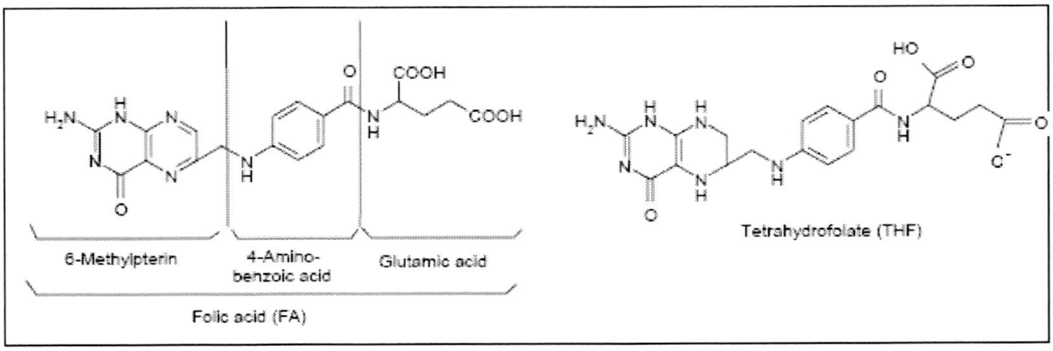

Figure 8.7.1. Formulas of folic acid (vitamin B11) and of tetrahydrofolate.

On the other hand it has been found, that vit.B11 exhibits a very strong cytostatic effect under the influence of ionizing radiation /7/. Experiments in vitro (using E.coli bacteria as a model) in aqueous media saturated with argon, air or N_2O, respectively, in order to generate diverse types of free radicals under gamma-ray treatment, were performed. The observed ΔD_{37}-data demonstrated the antitumor ability of vit.B11 under all conditions (Table 8.7.1.). The effect is depending on substrate concentration and on the dissolved gas. Hence, the highest ΔD_{37}-value was observed in airfree media. Comparable experiments with mitomycin C (MMC) showed, that e.g. $1x10^{-4}$ mol/L vit.B11 exhibits about the same cytostatic efficiency like $7.5x10^{-7}$ mol/L MMC. On the other hand by adding $5x10^{-5}$ mol/L vit.B11 to $7.5x10^{-7}$ mol/L MMC the activity of MMC was increased 2.5-times. This synergistic effect of vit.B11 is conducted to an electron transfer from the vitamin to MMC. This fact is obviously based on the $-NH_2$ and –NH– as well as on the –COOH groups contained in the FA-molecule, which are acting as electron donor /9/. Similar studies were also carried out at pH=6.2, where the observed ΔD_{37}(Gy)-values are found to be somewhat lower /7/.

It is further of interest to be mentioned, that the reactivity of vit.B11 with e_{aq}^- and OH is very high, namely: k (e_{aq}^- + FA) = 2.20 x 10^{10} L.mol $^{-1}$s $^{-1}$ and k (OH + FA) = 9.6 x 10^{9} L.mol $^{-1}$s $^{-1}$, respectively /8/. This fact indicates that the vitamine molecule can undergo decomposition, forming various products. Using 10^{-4} mol/L substrate in airfree media (pH = 7.4) the degradation yield was found to be the lowest one (G = 0.77), whereas in aerated solution, G = 1.83 and such saturated with N_2O was the highest one, G = 3.83 /7/. These results show, that the OH-radicals are the most successful species in the decomposition process.

Following this line of studies, several degradation products were established /7/. In airfree media a predominant formation of ammonia was found, which is mainly attributed to the attack of e_{aq}^- and H on the amino group. In addition a mixture of aldehydes was also determined. In media saturated with N_2O and especially in the presence of air, as main products of the oxidation reaction was found a mixture of carboxylic acids in addition to aldehydes. This is explainable by preferential OH-attack on the C=C and C=N double bonds in the vitamin molecule resulting into OH-adducts.

Table 8.7.1.: ΔD_{37}(Gy)-values*) of folic acid (FA) obtained from the corresponding survival curves in various media (pH=7.4) as well as of mitomycin C (MMC) individually and in mixture with FA /7/.

Substrate (mol/L)	ΔD_{37}(Gy)-values		
	Airfree 44% e_{aq}^-,10% H,46% OH	Aerated 46% OH, 54% $O_2^{\bullet -}$	N_2O 10% H, 90% OH
10^{-4} FA	-90	-40	-60
10^{-3} FA	-160	-60	-80
$7.5x10^{-7}$ MMC	-80	----	----
$7.5x10^{-7}$ MMC and $5x10^{-5}$ FA	-200	----	----

*) Negative ΔD37(Gy)-values indicate cytostatic ability of the substrate, whereas the positive ones, radiation protection

On the other hand the OH radicals can also split off a H-atom from the –NH– and $-NH_2$ groups etc., as well as abstract an electron from the substrate molecule. In general the resulting transients in the presence of air can add oxygen, resulting in very unstable peroxides, which lead to formation of aldehydes and carboxylic acids. Similary to OH, $O_2^{\bullet-}$ species in aerated solution can also attack the substrate, but much slower, giving rise to various final products.

In order to obtain a better insight in the reaction mechanisms initiatied by OH radicals, pulse radiolysis studies of vit.B11 were performed under appropriate conditions. Using 10^{-5} mol/L substrate in aqueous media (pH = 7.8), saturated with N_2O, where 90% OH and 10% H are operative, two transient absorption spectra were observed: A short-lived one (A) with λ_{max} = 425 nm (ε = 1.64 x 10^4 L.mol^{-1}cm^{-1}) and long lived (B) having λ_{max} = 335 nm (ε = 1.29 x 10^3 L.mol^{-1}cm^{-1}), which are shown in Figure 8.7.2. /10/.

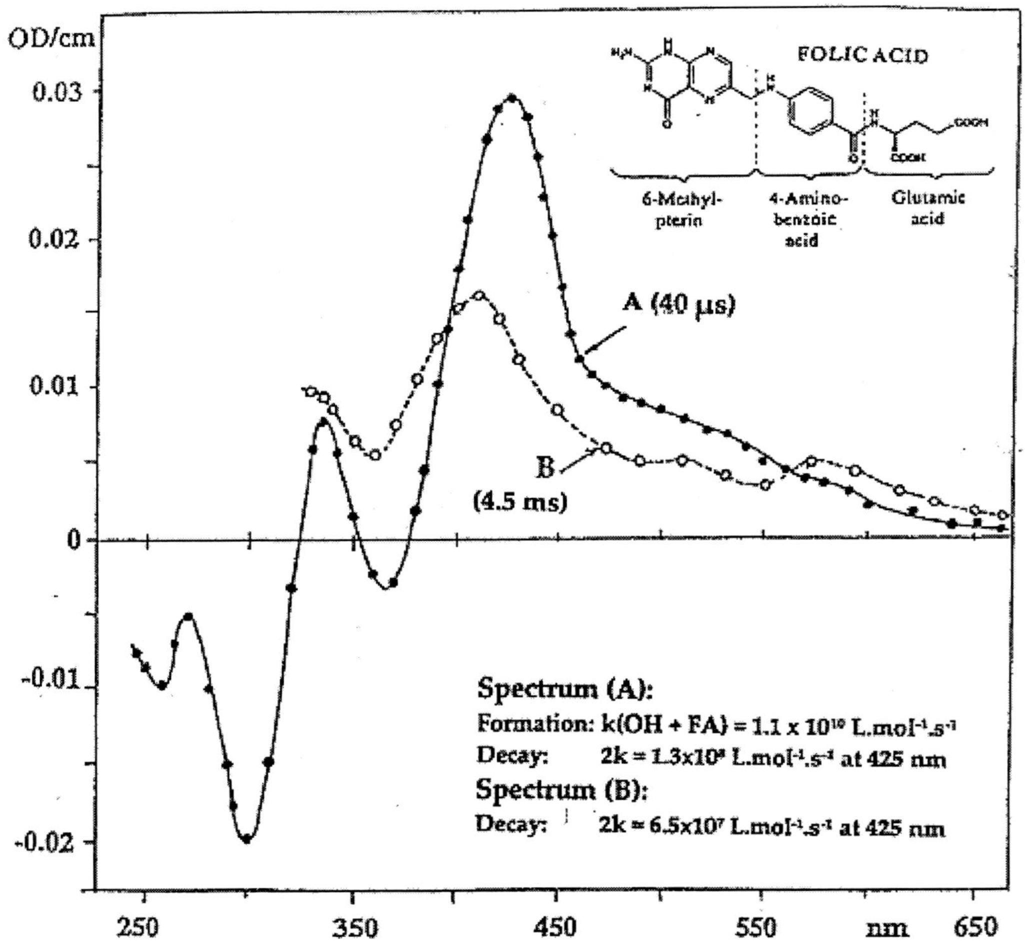

Figure 8.7.2. Transient absorption spectra observed by pulse radiolysis 1x10^{-5} mol/L folic acid in aqeous solution (pH=7.8) saturated with N_2O at: (A) 40-50 μs and (B) 4.3-4.8 ms after pulse, normalized to 10 Gy/pulse. (Reproduced with permission of Oncology Research, Vol.15, pp.295-300, 2005).

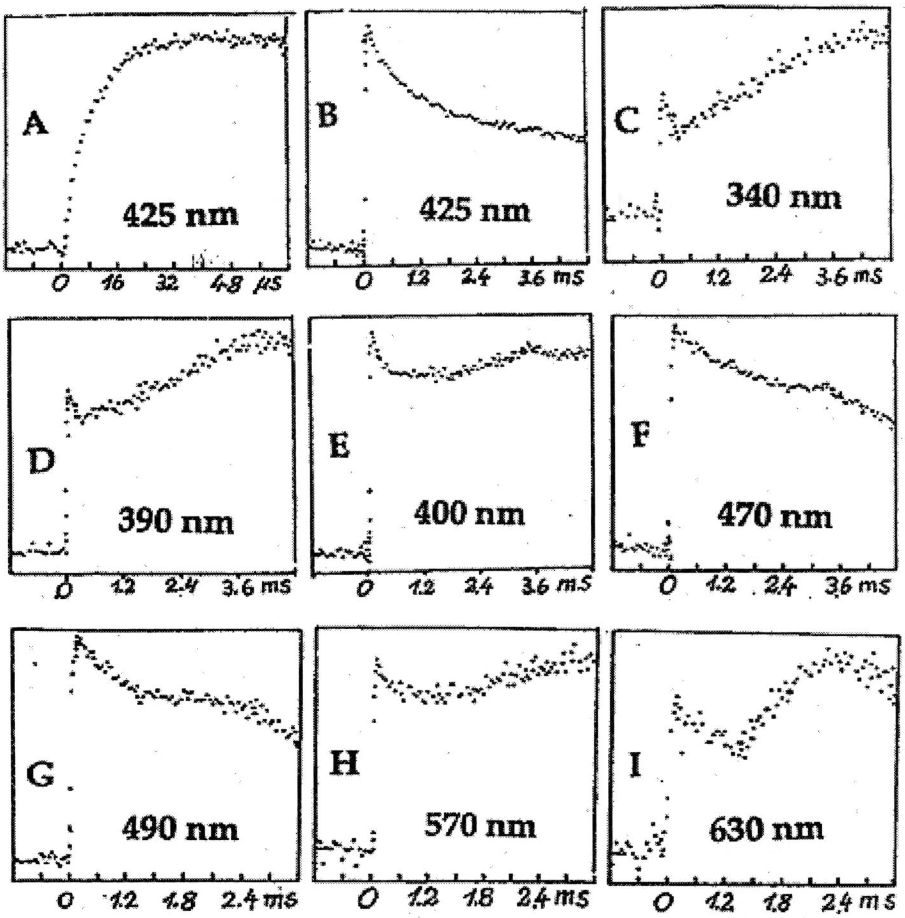

Figure 8.7.3. Kinetic profiles registered by OH attack on $1x10^{-5}$ mol/L FA in aqueous solutions saturated with N_2O (pH=7.8). (A) Formation and (B) decay of FA radicals at 425 nm (C–I) Kinetic traces showing the transformation of FA by intramolecular electron transfer process observed at various wavelengths. (Reproduced with permission of Oncology Research, Vol.15, pp.295-300, 2005).

Based on some preliminary calculations of the FA electronic structure, more than half a dozen transients should be formed by the OH attack on the substrate molecule. Hence, it is assumed that the expected transient absorption spectra are superimposed and cannot be resolved spectroscopically /10/.

Similar reaction mechanisms initiated by OH radicals on procarbacine were studied by two methods: pulse radiolysis and simulation computation (see chapter 4) /11/. For resolving of overlapping kinetic and spectroscopic data special computation method has been previously reported /12, 13/.

Following this line and based on the complex composition of the FA-molecule, studies of the formation and decay kinetics of FA-transients at various wavelengths were carried out. Some kinetic profiles (transient absorption as a function of time: µs, ms) were presented in Figure 8.7.3. From the formation and decay kinetics (A)- and (B)-profiles at the absorption maximum at 425 nm, the build-up rate constant, k(OH+FA) = 1.1×10^{10} $L.mol^{-1}s^{-1}$ and the bimolecular decay rate constant, 2k = 1.3×10^{8} $L.mol^{-1}s^{-1}$ at pH = 7.8 were determined. They are in good agreement with the previously reported ones /8/. The decay constant for spectrum (B) was 2k = 6.5 x 10 [7] L.mol $^{-1}$s $^{-1}$. On the other hand the kinetic profiles (C) to (I), Figure 8.7.3. show a peculiar course. Because the OH radicals are strongly electrophilic species, they attack specifically the most negative charged sites of the FA-molecule. The electronic stability of the first produced transients is based on the preceding negative charge force of the corresponding molecule site. Hence, FA-transients with different electronic stabilities (lifetimes) are formed, namely some with lower stability (very-short–lived) and others having more stable electron structure (longer-lived). Under such conditions the short lived transients tend to convert into more stable electron structures by intramolecular electron transfer. This process is for the first time registered on FA-transients as presented in Figure 8.7.3 /10/.

Naturally, the intramolecular electron transfer demonstrates a kind of "combat for electrons" within biological molecules, finally resulting into a longer-lived radical. This process is in competition with the reactivity towards adjacent molecules. Hence, the probability of causing a significant biological effect depends on the FA-radical concentration at the time of reaction on the specific rate constant (k-value) of the respective process.

It has been also reported that FA is used for the recovery of patients after therapy with methotrexate (MTX) /14, 15/. Further, it was found that folinic acid (FNA) is even more efficient in this respect than FA /16/. Since the chemical structures of FA, FNA and MTX are rather similar, their reaction rate constants with e_{aq}^- and OH were determined (Table 8.7.2) /10/.

Table 8.7.2.: Formulas of folic adic (FA), folinic acid (FNA) and methotrexate (MTX) as well as rate constants (k, L.mol $^{-1}$s $^{-1}$) for their reactions with e_{aq}^- and OH species. (Reproduced with permission of Oncology Research, vol.15, pp.295-300, 2005).

Formula	Rate constant (L.mol^{-1}.s^{-1})	
	k (e^-_{aq} + S)	k (OH + S)
FOLIC ACID 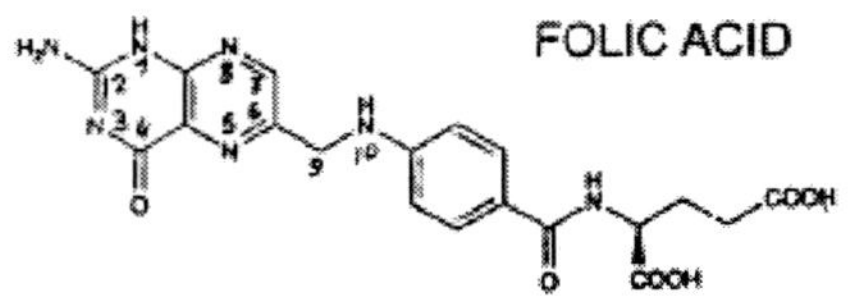	1.9 x 10^{10}	1.1 x 10^{10}
FOLINIC ACID 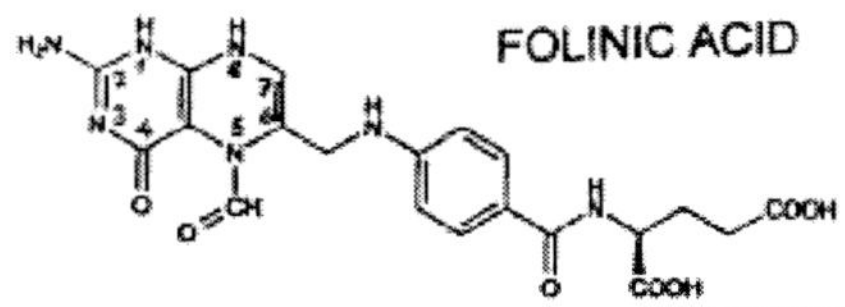	3.1 x 10^{10}	1.4 x 10^{10}
METHOTREXATE 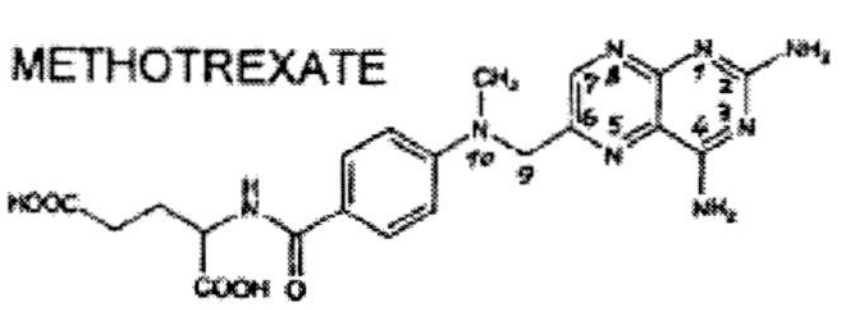	1.0 x 10^{10}	2.3 x 10^{10}

Comparing the kinetic values of the three compounds it is obvious that they are highly reactive with both, e_{aq}^- and OH, whereby the individual rate constants differentiate very slightly from each other, MTX has the lowest rate constant for the reaction with e_{aq}^-, however, the highest one for the OH-attack. Its structure shows two amino groups, on position 2 and 4; the reactive H atom on position 10 of FA and FNA molecules is replaced in MTX by the much less reactive $-CH_3-$group. Further, the amino groups in MTX may act as a source for electron ejection, when the molecule is excited in its single state /9/. In addition to this the amino groups are superior by their reactivity towards OH radicals. On the other side, the formyl group on position 5 of FNA molecule is responsible for its rather high rate constant for the reaction with e_{aq}^-. The electron affinity in such case is even stronger than that of halogen atoms incorporated in organic molecules /17/. This fact might explain why FNA supplementation in the frame of the MTX therapy is more efficient than FNA /16/. Based on this fact it can be assumed that an electron transfer form MTX (acting as electron donor) to FNA (electron acceptor) takes place (compare the $k(e_{aq}^- + S)$-values in Table 8.7.2.). From the kinetic data is obvious, that FNA seems to be a somewhat weaker electron acceptor than FNA. In reality the involved reaction mechanisms of these systems are certainly much more complicated, however, the proposed hypothesis may contribute to a better understanding of the involved processes.

8.7. References

[1] Roje, S., 2007, Vitamin B biosynthesis in plants. A review., Phytochem. 68, 1904-1921.

[2] Lucock, M. and Daskalakis, I., 2000, New perspectives on folate status: a differential role for the vitamin cardiovascular disease, birth defects and other conditions, *Br.J.Biomol.Sci.* 57, 254-260.

[3] Ratman, S.B., Delcamp, J.J., Hynes, J.B. and Freisheim, J.H., 1987, Purification and characterization of dihydrofolate reductase from soybean seedlings, *Arch.Biochem.Biophys.* 255, 279-289.

[4] Lazar, G. Toth, I., Haakonsen, L. and Goodman, H.M., 1989, Coregulation of dihydrofolate reductase and thymidylate synthese in overproducer cell lines of wild carrot, *Plan.Physiol.* 91, 1168-1173.

[5] Mohammad, A.M.S., Al-Chalabi, K. and Abood, S.A., 1989, Effect of folate analogues on the activity of dihydrofolate reductase and callus growth of sunflower, *J.Exp.ot.* 40, 701-706.

[6] Cella, R. and Parisi, B., 1993, Dihydrofolate reductase and thymidylate synthese in plants – an open problem, *Physiol.Plant* 88, 509-521.

[7] Delipetar-Grudl, A. and Getoff, N., 2004, Radiation-induced sensitizing effect of folic acid (vitamin B11) and its synergistic action to mitomycin C. In vitro experiments and radiolysis, *Oncology Res.* 14, 1607-1613.

[8] Moorthy, P.N. and Hayon, E., 1976, One electron redox reactions of water soluble vitamins. II. Pterin and folic acid, *J.Org.Chem.* 41, 1607-1613.

[9] Getoff, N, 1989, A review of the relationship between $Q(e_{aq}^-)$ and Q(F) of excited compounds in aqueous solution, *Radiat.Phys.Chem.* 34, 711-719.

[10] Getoff, N., 2005, Transient absorption spectra and kinetics of folic acid (vitamin B11) and some kinetic data of folinic acid and methotrexate, *Oncology Res.* 15, 295-300.
[11] Delipetar-Grudl, A., Solar, S. and Getoff, N., 2006, Reaction of OH-radicals with procarbacine. A pulse radiolysis and computer simulation study, *Anticancer Res.* 26, 405-410.
[12] Solar, S., Getoff, N., Solar, W. and Mark, F., 1981, A kinetic study of multiple H-attack on methylene blue in aqueous solution, *Radiat.Phys.Chem.* 17, 107-111.
[13] Solar, S., Solar, W. and Getoff, N., 1983, A semi-linear optimization model for resolving fast processes, *J.Chem.Soc.Faraday Trans.* 79, 123-135.
[14] Motycka, K. and Balcarova, A., 1975, Methotrexate and folic acid effect in normal sacoma 180 bearing mice, *Neoplasma* 22, 507-518.
[15] Guttormsen, A.B., Ueland, P.M., Loning, P.E., Mella, O. and Refsum, H., 2004, Inetics of plasma total homocystein in patients receiving high dose methotrexate therapy, *Clin.Chem.* 44, 1987-1989.
[16] Morgan, S.L., Oster, R.A., Lee, J.Y., Alarcoin, G.S. and Baggot, J.E., 2004, The effect of folinic acid supplements on purine metabolism in methotrexate-treated rheumatoid arthritis, *Arthritis Rheum.* 50, 3104-3111.
[17] Solar, S., Getoff, N., Holcman, J. and Sehested, K., 1995, Radical anions of chlorinated benzaldehydes in aqueous solution, *J.Phys.Chem.* 99, 9425-9429.

8.8. Vitamin B12 (Cyanocobalamin)

Vitamin B12 (vit.B12, Cyanocobalamin; 5,6-dimethyl-benzimidazolyl-cyanocobamide) known also under various names is prototype of the family of naturally occurring cobalt coordination compounds, called corrinoids. The richest source of vit.B12 is activated sewage sludge. It is also contained in meat, liver and fish, however plants have very little or no cobalamins. Vit.B12 consists of hygroscopic, dark red crystals and is water soluble. Its formuma is rather complicated (Figure 8.8.1.), having various functional groups and therefore many-sided biological properties.

Vitamin B12 is frequently used in combination with other B-vitamins in complex and helps to maintain healthy nerve cells and red blood cells, and is implemented in DNA synthesis. Since the human body stores vit.B12 for years, nutritional deficiency of this vitamin is rather rare /1/. However, an eventual vit.B12 deficiency can lead to neurology symptoms, muscle weakness, incontinence, hypotension vision problems, dementia and psychoses. People at risk for vit.B12 deficiency include vegetarians, elderly people and such with increased requirements associated with pregnancy, haemolytic anemia, malignancy, liver and kidney diseases. It was found, that patients diagnosed with Alzheimer´s disease have abnormally low vit.B12 levels in their blood /2/. The lack of vit.B12 is also associated with various kinds of cancer /3-7/. On the other hand it has been observed, that patients with average age of 74,4 years the length of survival decreased with the increase in serum vitamin B12 levels (P = 0.0015, Cox model). This data indicated, that an elevated serum vitamin B12 level is a predictive factor for mortality in patients with cancer /8/.

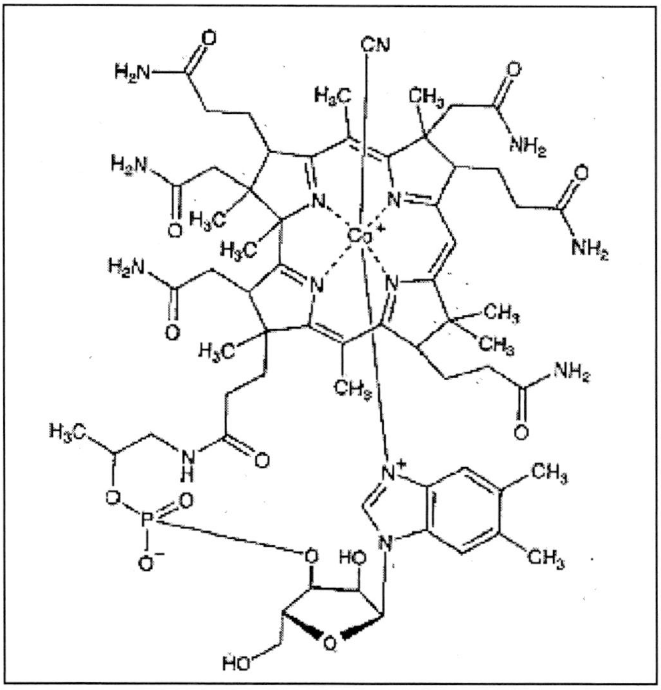

Figure 8.8.1. Structure formula of vitamin B12.

On the other hand it has been found, that vitamin B12 in combination with other vitamins, particularly with vitamin B11 (folic acid) exhibits antitumor effect, cancer prevention as well as positive effect in radiation treatment of cancer /9-13/. The combined implementation of vitamin B11 (folic acid) and vitamin B12 was found to decrease hip fracture risk in elderly people with stroke /14/.

Finally, it can be stated, that although an abundant literature reports about versatile biological effects of vitamin B12, implemented individually or in combination with other vitamins and related compounds, practically nothing is known about the involved reaction mechanisms. On the other hand, however, based on its moleculare structure (see Figure 8.8.1.), one can deduce, that e.g. the available –OH and -NH_2 substituents can emit electrons, whereas the –CO group can scavange electrons /15/. Hence, vitamin B12 can act as an efficient electron mediator , depending on the involved redox-systems. Starting from this postulation one can explain at least some of the observed effects by electron transfer from vitamin B12 to an appropriate partner, or opposite vitamin B12 scavenges electrons ejected e.g. from vitamin B11 (folic acid), enzymes etc. Investigations in this respect could contribute to a better understanding of the subject matter and perhaps to an improvement of cancer prevention or/and treatment.

8.8. References

[1] Lindenbaum, J., Healton, E.B., Savage, D.G. et. al., 1988, Neuropsychiatric disorders caused by cobalamin deficiency in the asence of anemia or macrocytosis, New *Engl.J.Med.* 318, 1720-1728.

[2] McCaddon, A. and Kelly, C.L., 1994, Familial Alzheimer′s disease and vitamin B12 deficiency, Age and Ageing 23, 2334-337.

[3] Schreurs, W.H., Oddink, J., Egger, R.J., Wedel, M. and Bruning, P.F., 1985, The influence of radiotherapy and chemotherapy on the vitamin status of cancer patients, *Int.J.Vitam.Nutr.Res.* 55, 425-432.

[4] Kato, H., Hirano, T., Shibanuma, H., Okada, S., Saito, M. and Konaka, C. 1995, Reevaluation of preneoplastic lung lesions in lung carcinoma? In bronchial carcinoma?, Can.To Kagaku Ryoho 22, 2048-2054.

[5] Choi, Sang-Woon, 1999, Vitamin B12 deficiency: A new risk factor for breast cancer?, *Nutrition Rev.* 57, 250-260.

[6] Wu, K. et al., 1999, A prospective study of folate, B12 and pyridoxal-5`-phosphate (B6) and breast cancer, *Cancer Epidem.Biomark.Prev.* 8, 209-217.

[7] Hartman, P.J., Woodson, K., Stolzenberg-Solomon, R. et al., 2001, Association of the B-vitamins pyrdoxal 5′-phosphate (B6) and folate with lung cancer risk in older man, *Am.J.Epidemiol.* 153, 688-694.

[8] Geissbühler, Ph., Bernadette, M. and Rapin, Ch.-H., 2000, Elevated serum vitamin B12 levels associated with CRP as a predicative factor of mortality in palliative care cancer patients: A prospective study over five years, *J.Pain and Sympt.Mang*. 20, 93-103.

[9] Levitman, M.Kh., Kublik, L.N., Shaposhnikova, V.V., Akatov, V.S. and Korystov, Iu.N., 2002, Antitumor effect of combined treatment with ionizing radition and vitamin B12 complex, *Radiat.Biol.Radioecol.*(Russ.) 42, 511-514.

[10] Tsuchida, T., Saito, M., Honda, H., Hirata, T. and Kato, H., 2003, Chemoprevention of lung cancer, Gan To Kagaku Ryoho 30, 181-184.

[11] Zhang, S.M., 2004, Role of vitamins in the risk, prevention and treatment fo breast cancer, *Curr.Opin.Obsted.Gynecol.* 16, 19-25.

[12] Branda, R.F., Nand, S.J., Brooks, E.M., Chen, Z. and Muss, H., 2004, Effect of vitamin B12, folate and dietary supplements on breast carcinoma chemotherapy–induced mucositis and neutropenia, *Cancer* 101, 1058-1064.

[13] Kapiszewska, M., Kalemba, M., Wojciech, U. and Milewicz, T., 2005, Uracil misincorporation into DNA of leucocytes of young women with positive folate balance depends on plasma vitamin B12 concentrations and methylenetetrahydrofolate reductase polymorphisms. A pilot study, J.Nation.Biochem. 16, 467-478.

[14] Uebelhart, B. and Rizzoli, R., 2006, Osteoporosis treatment, *Rev.Med.Suisse* 2, 47-51.

[15] Getoff, N., 2007, Anti-aging and aging factors in life. The role of free radicals, *Radiat.Phys.Chem.* 76, 1577-1586.

Chapter 9

Other Vitamins of Interest

9.1. Vitamin A (Retinol)

Vitamin A (Vit.A; retinol; all-trans retinol; 3,7-dimethyl-9-(2,6,6-trimethyl-1-cyclohexen-1-yl)-2,4,6,8-nonatetraethyl-1-ol; anti-infective vitamin) occurs in animals, but not in plants. The symmetric oxidative cleavage of the carotenoid molecule results into retinal, which is converted into retinol (vitamin A) by the liver (Figure 9.1.1.).

Vitamin A is a growth vitamin having various biological properties. It is also involved in the rather complex vision process. The light sensitive dye-pigment of the eye, rhodopsin consists mainly of the protein opsin and neoretinol b, a stereoisomere of all-trans-retinol (vitamin A aldehyde), which mediates the visionary power.

An excellent overview about the various aspects concerning vitamin A, such as its biological functions, methods of nutritional assessment, factors influencing the vitamin status, hazards of high dose use etc. are discussed by Olsons /1/. In addition to determining the relative biological activity of vitamin A, also cell and organ culture systems were used for studies. The aim was to gain an insight into the mechanisms by which retinoids induce differentiation of cells and prevent the development of neoplastic cells.

Concerning the efficiency of all-trans retinoic acid (RA) and interferon-α (IFN-α) on premalignant and malignant models of cervical cancers it was found /2/.: (i) using RA the cell growth rate was inhibited to 84-96% in human papilloma-virus type 18 (HPV18)-immortilized endocervical cells as well as for SiHa abd ME 180 cells, but 18-62% for other cells. (ii) By IFN-α about 75% in SiHa and Me180 as well as 14-40% in other cell lines.

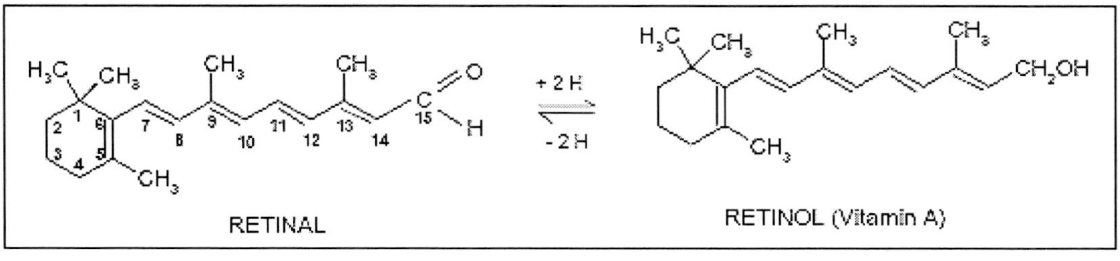

Figure 9.1.1. Structure formulas of retinal and retinol.

Combining RA and IFN-α increased the antiproliferative effect in premalignant and some other cancer cells, except SiHa, OMC-4 and HT-3 cells. These results show that the inhibition of cell growth by RA and IFN-α depends on: cell origin, cell line, oncology state as well as on treatment type and time.

In a recent review, the key role of naturally occurring retinols and their analogies in cell differentiation, proliferation and apoptosis and their potential use in oncology, dermatology and in variety of diseases are discussed /3/. Thereby the role of vitamin A and its metabolism in oncology and dermatology has been successfully used in differentiated therapy of acute promicelocytic leukaemia, skin cancer, etc. and in treatment of acne and psoriasis. Its usefulness is, however, limited by the rapid emergence of acquired vitamin A resistance, based on a multifactor mechanism. One possible pathway to overcome this limitation was to inhibit the action of the cytochrome P450-dependent vitamin A-4-hydroxylase enzymes (particularly CYP26b) responsible for vitamin A metabolism.

The action mechanism of retinoids, retinoic acids and receptors are still not completely understood, hence further studies in this respect are desirable.

9.1. References

[1] Olson, J.A., 1990, Vitamin A, pp. 1-57 in "Handbook of Vitamins", ed. Machlin L.J., Publ. Marcel Dekker, Inc., New York, Basel

[2] Yokoyama, M., Nakao, Y., Iwasaka, T., Pater, A. and Sugimori, H., 2001, Retinoic acid and interferon-α effects on cell growth and differentiation in cervical cell lines, Amer.College of Obstetricians and Gynecologists, 98, 332-???

[3] Njar, V.C.U., Gediya, L., Purushotramachar, P. et al., 2006, Retinoic acid metabolism blocking agents for treatment of cancer and dermatological diseases, *Bioorganic and Med.Chem.* 14, 4323-4340.

9.2. Biotin (Vitamin H)

Bitotin (vitamin H; hexahydro-2-oxo-1H-thieno[3,4-id]imidazole-4-pentanoic acid; cis-hexahydro-2-oxo-1H-thieno[3,4]-imidazole-4-valeric acid; coenzyme R; biodermatin) is a growth factor present in every living cell. It occurs mainly bound to proteins and polypeptides and plays a role in various naturally occurring carboxylation processes. The richest sources are liver, kidney, pancreas, yeast and milk. The biotin content in cancer cells is higher than that of normal ones. The vitamin properties of biotin become inactivated by bonding to the protein avidin (see also Fig. 9.2.1.).

In the frame of an extensive report the chemistry, biochemical functions, metabolism, nutrition requirements and efficiency of pharmacological doses of biotin have been discussed /1/.

Biotin serves in mammals as a coenzyme for acetyl-CoA carboxylase, pyruvat carboxylase, propionyl-CoA carboxylase and 3-methylcrotonyl-CoA carboxylase. Based on its many-sided functions, it has been observed, that biotin deficiency may enhance the resistance of cancer cells to antineoplastic agents /2/.

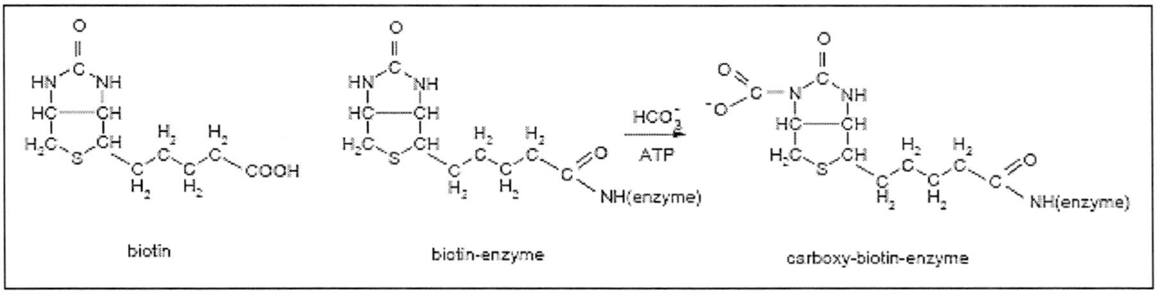

Figure 9.2.1. Structure formulas of biotin, biotin-enzyme and carboxy-biotin-enzyme.

On the other hand, because of the high affinity of biotin for proteins and related compounds it was implemented as cancer-cell targeting vehicle that can deliver biotinylated therapeutic drugs /e.g.3/. In addition to this, biotin as well as some of its derivatives were labelled with radionucleids and used for targeted radiotherapy of cancer /4/, as well as for prolonged drug delivery in respect to ovarian cancer /5/. In this case the use of avidin-biotin liposome system (^{9m}Tc-labelled) was investigated /6/.

9.2. References

[1] BIOTIN; Jean-Pierre Bonjour, pp. 394-427 in "Handbook of Vitamins", ed. L.J.Machlin, Marcel Dekker, Inc., New York, Basel (1990).

[2] Griffin, J.B. and Zempleni, J., 2005, Biotin deficiency stimulates survival pathways in human lymphoma cells exposed to antineoplastic drugs, *J.Nutrit.Biochem.* 16, 96-103.

[3] Wilbur, D.S., Panthhare, P.M., Hamlin, D.K. et al., 1999, Development of new biotin-streptavidin reagents for pretargeting, *Biomol.Engin.* 16, 113-116.

[4] Lewis, M.R., Zhang, J., Jia, F., Owen, N.K. et al., 2004, Biological comparison ^{149}Pm, ^{166}Ho and ^{177}Lu-DOTA-biotin pretargeted by CC49 scF-streptavidin fusion protein in xeno-graft bearing nude mice, *Nucl.Med.Biol.* 31, 213-223.

[5] Grana, Ch., Bartolomei, M., Handkeiwicz, D., Rocca, P. et al., 2004, Radioimmuntherapy in advanced ovarian cancer: is there a role for pre-targeting with ^{90}Y-biotin?, *Ginecol.Oncology* 93, 691-698.

[6] Zavaleta, C.L., Phillips, W.T. et al., 2007, Use of avidin-biotin-liposome system for enhanced peritoneal drug delivery in an ovarian cancer model. *Int.J.Pharmaceutics* 337, 316-328.

9.3. Vitamin D

The designation vitamin D embraces a group of related compounds having anti-rachiting activity, namely: vitamin D1 (mol.wt. 793,3), vitamin D2 (3β, 5Z, 7E, 22E)-9,10-Secoergosta-5-7,10(19)22-teraen-3-ol, calciferol, ergocalciferol, activated ergosterol; mol.wt. 396,66), vitamin D3 (3β, 5Z, 7E)-9,10-Secoergosta-5-7,10-(19)-terien-3-ol; activated 7-dehydrocholesterol; cholecalciferol, delosterol; mol.wt. 384,65) and vitamin D4 ((3β, 5Z,

7E)-9,10-Secoergosta-5-7,10(19)- trien-3-ol; 22:23-di-hydrovitamin D2; dihydrocalciferol; mol.wt. 398,67). The most prominent members of the group are: (i) vitamin D2, which is derivated from a common plant steroid (ergosterol) and is usually employed for vitamin D in foods. (ii) Vitamin D3 obtained by conversion of the precursor, 7-dehydrocholesterol, under the influence of sunlight on skin. Hence, vitamin D is also designated as prohormone, metabolized to a biologically active form that acts as a steroid hormone. Vitamin D, together with two peptide hormones (calcitonin and parathyroid) plays an important role in phosphorins homeostasis, where phosphorous and calcium are required for great variety of biological processes. Phosphorous is needed e.g. for genetic information (DNA and RNA), membrane structures, enzyme-protein components, phospholipids etc., whereas calcium is necessary for muscle contraction, nerve pulse transmission, membrane structure and blood clotting. Both, calcium and phosphorous are very important for the bone mineralization (tricalcium phosphate).

The structure formulas of the vitamins D2, D3 and D4 are presented in Figure 9.3.1. for information.

It should be noted that vitamin D has to be first metabolized to its most active forms, $1,25(OH)_2D_3$, before it can exhibit any biological function. This process takes place in the liver and is catalized by the enzyme vitamin D-23-hydroxylase, involving the addition of a OH-group on the 25-carbon. Therefore, the level of $25(OH)D_3$ is a good index of vitamin D status. The $25(OH)D_3$ is then transported from the liver to the kidney, where a second OH-group is added at the C-1 position, resulting into the very active $1,25(OH)_2D_3$ form /1/. The production of the hormone $1,25(OH)_2D_3$ can be modulated according to the calcium needs of the organism. A second dihydroxylated metabolite of vitamin D is produced in the kidney, namely $24,25(OH)_2D_3$. The responsible enzyme in this case is the 25-hydroxyvitamin-D_3-4-hydroxylase (24-hydroxylase). The activity of this enzyme is regulated: when $1,25(OH)_2D_3$ levels are low, the activity of 24-hydroxylase is also low and reverse. There is also evidence that $24,25(OH)_2D_3$ among other activities is involved in the mineralization of bone. In addition to this it appears that the combined action of both, $1,25(OH)_2D_3$ and $24,25(OH)_2D_3$, may be required for some of the known biological processes of vitamin D.

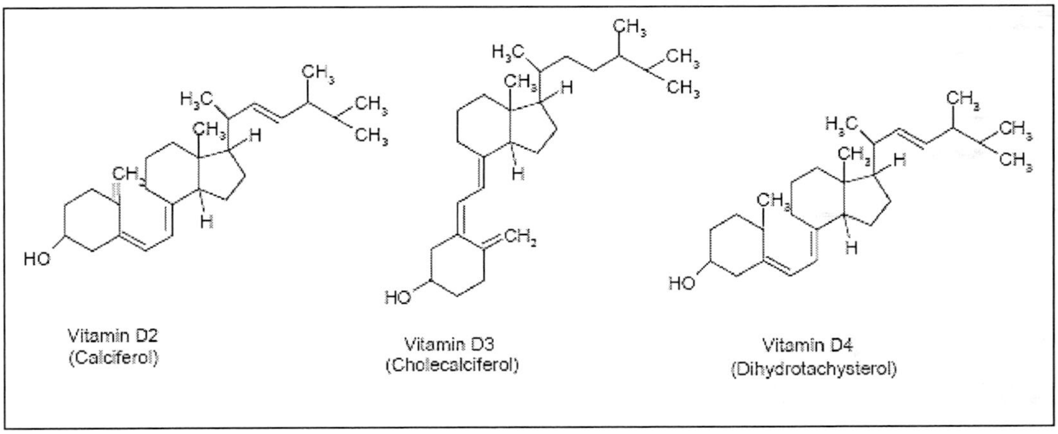

Figure 9.3.1. Structure formulas of vitamin D2, D3 and D4.

It should be also noted, that in addition to the above mentioned D_3-metabolites the existence of about 30 other metabolites are known. Most of them appear to be intermediates of the degradation pathway of $1,25(OH)_2D_3$.

It has been reported that especially $1,25(OH)_2D_3$ and $24,25(OH)_2D_3$ structures play a determining role in respect to prevention and therapy of cancer. $1,25(OH)_2D_3$, the hormonally active metabolite of vitamin D3, can influence several biological processes: cellular growth, differentiation and function not only in intestine, kidney and bone, but also in a large number of tissues and various cell types. It can also suppress the growth of malignant tissues or cancer cell lines, e.g. osteosarcoma, mycloid and lymphocytic leukaemia, cervical and breast carcinoma /2-6/. It has also been shown that $1,25(OH)_2D_3$ is a rather potent inhibitor of malignant growth of human colon adenocarcinoma-derived Caco-2 cells /7/. In addition to metabolizing $1,25(OH)_2D_3$ along the C-24 and C-23 oxidative pathways, Caco-2 cells are able to synthesize $1,25(OH)_2D_3$ from $25(OH)D_3$ through constitutive expression of $25(OH)D_3$-1α-hydroxlase activity /8/.

It is further observed, that during the progression of colon tumour cells the enzyme CyP27B1, which is essential for the $1,25(OH)_2D_3$ synthesis, as well as vitamin D receptor (VDR) appear at higher levels. This effect results in a physiological defence against tumour progression /9/. On the other hand a significant correlation between low exposure to sunlight in Scandinavian countries and an incidence of mammary, prostate and colorectal cancer has been established /10/. The consumption of oily fish by the population in northern countries keeps the level of 25-D_3 serum about normal. However, low levels of 25-D_3-serum is correlated to incidence of prostate cancer /11/. With the realization of external synthesis and degradation of $1,25(OH)_2D_3$ a link to low serum levels of $1,25(OH)_2D_3$ to prostate cancer was established /12/.

It should be mentioned, that also in USA the highest colon cancer mortality was observed in the population less exposed to solar irradiation, since UV-B is responsible for the production of vitamin D in the skin /13/. Low levels of $25(OH)D_3$-serum were found in African-Americans, probably as a reduction of vitamin D synthesis as a consequence of the high melanin concentration in the skin. This population showed an enhanced incidence of colorectal, breast and prostate cancer /14/.

A number of these studies were also concerned with the role of population nutrition in addition to the vitamin D and calcium consumption in respect to the observed effects. An excellent overview about vitamin D and its various biological effects as well as in the prevention of cancer is presented recently by Cross /15/.

The briefly presented survey demonstrates the many-sided biological importance of vitamin D. However, nothing is known about the action of free radicals on vitamin D, in respect to its generation, biological efficiency and metabolism. The UV-B part of the sunlight, needed for the synthesis of vitamin D can also initiate a number of photo-biological processes in the skin. In addition to generation of "solvated electrons" (e_{aq}^-; the basic form of H atoms) it can also lead to the formation of various types of free radicals. Therefore, in order to get a better understanding of the involved processes initiated by sunlight, specific designed studies are urgently needed. On the other hand, human organism is continuously producing and consuming oxidizing (e.g. OH, $O_2^{\bullet -}$ etc.) and reducing free radicals (e_{aq}^-, $R^\bullet$ etc.), which are implemented in numerous biological processes it is unavoidable, that these intermediates should react with vitamin D as well as with its precursors and metabolites. Investigations in this respect will essentially contribute for the understanding of the involved reaction mechanisms.

9.3. References

[1] Machlin L-J., ed., "Handbook of vitamins"; Marcel Dekker, Inc., New York, Basel (1990)

[2] De Luca H.F., Ostrem V., 1986, The relationship between vitamin D system and cancer, Adv.Exp.Med.Biol. 206, 413-429.

[3] Studzinski G.P., McLane J.A., Uskokovic M.R., 1993, Signaling pathways for vitamin D-induced differentiation. Implications for therapy of proliferative and neoplastic diseases, Crit.Rev.*Eukaryot.Gene Expr.* 3, 279-312.

[4] Cross H.S., Pavelka M., Slavik J., Peterlik M., 1992, Growth control of human colon cancer cells by vitamin D and calcium in vitro, *J.Natl.Cancer Inst.* 84, 1355-1357.

[5] Cross H.S., Farsondi K.H., Peterlik M., 1993, Growth inhibition of human colon adenocarcinoma-derived Caco-2 cells by 1α, 2S$(OH)_2D_3$ and two synthetic analogues. Relation to in vivo hypercalcemic potential, Naunyn-Schmiedbergs *Arch.Pharmacol.* 347, 105-110.

[6] Reichrath J., Friedrich M., Tilgen W. (eds.), 2003, Vitamin D Analogues in Cancer Prevention and Therapy, Springer, Berlin, Heidelberg.

[7] Giuliano A.R., Franceschi T.R., Wood R.J., 1991,Characterization of the vitamin D receptor from the Caco-2 human colon carcinoma cell line. Effect of cellular differentiation, *Arch.Biochem.Biophys.* 285, 261-269.

[8] Cross H.S., Peterlik M., Reddy G.S., Schuster I., 1997, Vitamin D metabolism in human colon adenocarcinoma-derived Caco-2 cells. Expression of 25-hydroxy vitamin D_3-1α-hydroxylase activity and regulation of side-chain metabolism, *J.Steroid.Biochem.Molec.Biol.* 62, 21-28.

[9] Cross H.S., Kallay E., Farhan H., Weiland T.m Manhart T., 2003, Regulation of external vitamin D metabolism as a tool for colon and prostata prevention.pp. 413-425 in "Vitamin D Analogues in Cancer Prevention and Therapy", eds. Reichrat J., Friderich M., Tilgen W., Springer, Berlin, Heidelberg, 2003.

[10] Grant W.B., 2002, An estimate of premature cancer mortality in the United States due to inadequate doses of solar ultraviolet-B-radiation, *Cancer* 94, 1867-1875.

[11] Tuohima P., Lyakhovich A., Aksenov N., Pennanem P., et al., 2001, Vitamin D and prostate cancer, *J.Steroid.Biochem.Mol.Biol.* 76, 125-134.

[12] Schwarz G.G., Whitlatch L.W., Chen T.C. et al., 1998, Human prostate cells scynthezise 1,2,5-dihydroxyvitamin D_3 from 25-hydroxyvitamin D, Cancer Epidemiol. *Biomarkers Prev.* 7, 391-395.

[13] Tangpricha V., Pearce E.N., Chen T.C., Holick M.F., 2002, Vitamin D insufficiency among free living healthy young adults, *Amer.J.Med.* 112, 659-662.

[14] Freedman D.M., Dosemeci M., Mc.Glynn K., 2002, Sunlight and mortality from breast, ovarian, colon, prostate and nonmelanoma skin cancer. A composite dead certificate based case-control study, Occup.Environ.Med. 59, 257-262.

[15] Cross H.S., Vitamin D and colon cancer, pp.1709-1725, in "Vitamin D", 2nd edition, eds. Feldman F., Pike J.W., Glorieux et al., Academic Press Inc., San Diego, 2005.

Chapter 10

Further Antitumor Compounds

In addition to the above discussed antitumor systems there is a number of further compounds showing the same properties. In this respect just two of them, inositol and aspirin, are very briefly mentioned.

10.1. Inositol

Inositol has been isolated from muscle by Scherer (1850). It is existing in nine isomers, but just one of them, myoinositol (Cis-1,2,3,5-trans-4,6-cyclohexane-hexol) is biologically active (Figure10.1).

Actually, inositol appears in the nature as hexaphosphoric acid and is most frequently bonded on various metal ions, such as calcium, magnesium, iron, sodium etc. The Ca-Mg-inositol hexaphosphate (IP6; Figure10.1) is the most abundant form of this biologically very efficient compound.

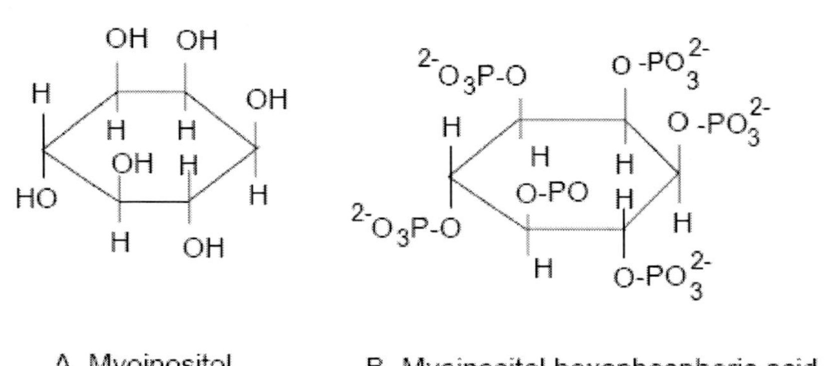

Figure 10.1. Formulas of biological active forms of inositol. (A) Myoinositol and (B) Myoinositol hexaphosphoric acid.

It is contained in various nutrients, such as: corn (~ 6 %), sesame (~ 5.7 %), wheat (1-5 %), beans (~ 2.5 %), rice (~ 2.2 %), peanuts (~ 2 %), soy beans (upto 1.8 %) etc. It has been established that IP6 has a rather broad spectrum of biological properties, first of all in respect to prevention and treatment of cancer, osteoporosis, diabetes, heart disease as well as depression /1-6/.

It has been observed, that over 99 % of the ingested IP6 in humans is reduced upto less than 50 % by dietary consume of calcium /2/.

As already indicated IP6 is successfully implemented in the last decades for cancer prevention and therapy. There are more than 27.000 published papers in this respect /3/, concerning various kinds of cancer /see e.g.7-13/.

At the present state of knowledge it is recommendable to employ the best modern pharmaceutical as well as naturopathic medical approaches, and if necessary, also combination of both, for the treatment of patients suffering on cancer. This suggestion is based on the fact, that the immuno-system of patients as well as the behaviour against drugs is rather individual in addition to the various stages of the sickness.

10.1. References

[1] Ishikava T. Ogawa S., Shamsuddin A.K.M., 2005; editors, Special Issue of Anticancer Research on: Desease prevention by IP6 and other rice components, *Anticancer Res.*19, No.5A, 3633-3791.

[2] Cody M.M., 1990, Substances without vitamin status, pp. 565-582 in Handbook of Vitamins (2nd edition) ed.by Machlin L.J.; Marcel Dekker Inc. New York.

[3] Vanderlinden K. and Vucenik J., 2004, Inositol + Ca Mag IP6. To good to be true. Prevention and treatment of: cancer, osteoporosis, depression, diabetes, heart disease and more, published by Bearing Marketing Comm.Ltd., Canada.

[4] Informatics, Inc., 1973, Scientific Literature Reviews on Generally Recognized as Safe (GRAS) Food Ingredients – Inositol, NTIS No. PB223861

[5] 1978, Inositol: Proposed Affirmation of GRAS status as a direct Human Food Ingredient, Federal Register, 43, 22056-22058.

[6] Baten A., Tomazic V.J. and Shamasuddin A.M., 1989, Inositol-phosphate induced enhancement of natural diller cell activity correlates with tumor suppression, *Carcinogenesis* 10, 1595-1598.

[7] Burkitt D.P., 1971, Epidemiology of cancer of the colon and rectum, Cancer 28, 3-13.

[8] Chatenoud L., Tavani A., La Vecchia C. et al., 1998, Whole grain food intake and cancer risk. *Intern.J.Cancer* 77, 24-28.

[9] Deliers L.G., Servida G. et al., Effects of inositol hexaphosphate (IP6) on human normal and leukaemic hematopoietic cells, *Brit.J.Haematology* 117, 577-578.

[10] DeStefani E., Correa P. et al., 1997, Dietary fiber and risk of breast cancer. A case control study in Uruguay, *Nutrition and Cancer* 28, 14-19.

[11] Hill M.J., Cereals, cereal fibre and colorectal cancer risk: A review of the epidemiological literature, *Europ.J.Cancer Prev.*6, 219-225.

[12] Grases F., Simonet B.M., Vucenik J. et al., 2001, Absorption and excretion of orally administrated inositol hexaphosphate (IP6 or phytate) in humans, *Bio Factors* 15, 53-61.

[13] Grases F., Simonet B.M., Vucenik J. et al., 2002, Effects of exogenous inostiol hexaphosphate (IP6) on inositol triphosphate (IP3) and IP6 in malignant cells, tissues and biological fluids, *Life Sciences* 71, 1533-1546.

10.2. Aspirin

Aspirin (Asp., salicylic acid acetate) is one of the most frequently used pharmaceutics. Its various biological properties and toxicity as well as clinical trials have been previously reported /1-3/. It has been also indicated, that aspirin is a rather efficient scavenger of free radicals, having rate constants for reaction with e_{aq}^{-}, k ≈ 10^{10} $L.mol^{-1}s^{-1}$, with H-atoms, k ≈ 2 x 10^{9} $L.mol^{-1}s^{-1}$ and with OH-radicals, k ≈ 1.5 x 10^{10} $L.mol^{-1}s^{-1}$ /19/. The aspirin formula is given in Figure 10.2.

Experiments in vitro, using Escherichia coli bacteria (AB1157) as a model, demonstrated, that aspirin shows well pronounced cytostatica effect. Moreover, aspirin can strongly influence the antitumor activity of mitomycin C (MMC) in dependence of the kind of free radicals involved in the system (see Table 10.2) /4/.

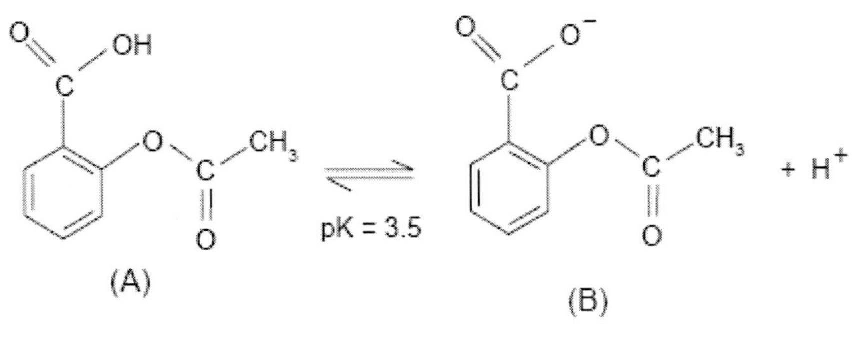

Figure 10.2. Protonated (A) and unprotonated form (B) of aspirin. Form (B) is biologically active.

The data in Table 10.2 clearly demonstrate that aspirin in all media (attack by oxidizing or/and reducing free radicals) shows a rather strong antitumor effect in comparison to that of MMC. It is interesting to state, that the mixtures of aspirin and MMC in aerated (A) and airfree (B) media exhibit lower ΔD_{37}-values, indicating protecting properties of aspirin (see the above reaction rate constants). However, in media (C) saturated with N_2O, the antitumor efficiency of aspirin (ΔD_{37} = - 65) as well as this of MMC (ΔD_{37} = - 105) and that of mixture of both substrates (ΔD_{37} = - 180) show a rather high antitumor efficiency. This also indicates the appearance of a synergistic effect of aspirin towards MMC.

The observed results refer to the involvement of multi-layer reaction mechanisms, which are presently not clear.

Table 10.2. ΔD_{37}-values derived from survival curves (N/N_0-ratio) as a function of absorbed radiation dose (Gy) of E.coli bacteria (AB1157) in buffered aqueous media containing 5×10^{-5} mol/L aspirin and 2.5×10^{-6} mol/L MMC and mixture of both at pH = 7.4; where: $\Delta D_{37} = D^0_{37} - D^s_{37}$; D^0_{37} = radiation dose of (Gy) of buffer at $N/N_0 = 0.37$; D^s_{37} = radiation dose of (Gy) of sample at $N/N_0 = 0.37$. The positive ΔD_{37}-values indicate protection from free radical attack (radiation protection), the negative ΔD_{37}-values demonstrate the antitumor effect of the system

System	ΔD_{37}(Gy) - values		
	A. Air 54% $O_2^{\bullet -}$, 46% OH	B. Argon 44% e_{aq}^-, 10% H, 46% OH	C. N_2O 90% OH, 10% H
Aspirin	- 60	- 25	- 65
MMC	- 95	- 90	- 105
Asp.+ MMC	- 80	- 55	- 180

10.2. References

[1] Smith M.J.H. and Smith P.K., 1966, The salicylates, Interscience Publ.Comp., New York.

[2] Barnett H.J.M. et al., 1982, Acetylsalicylic acid, Raven Publ.Comp., New Yyork.

[3] Proceed.Symp. on Aspirin Therapy, 1983, *Am.J.Med.*74, 1-109.

[4] Kammerer C. and Getoff N., 2001, Cytostatica action of aspirin and ist effect on mitomycin C activity. A study in vitro under irradiation, *Radiat.Phys.Chem.*61, 35-40.

Chapter 11

Sexual Hormones and Cancer

General Remarks

Hormones are biological substances, produced in human and animal organisms by endocrine glands and specific tissues. Although generated in very low concentration they show very specific biological actions by controlling important processes in the organism. The number of natural hormones generated in organism can be divided into: (i) steroid hormones, (ii) hormones derived from amino acids and (iii) peptid- and proteohormones /1/. In addition to these groups the phytohormones, contained in plants, become of great interest in medicine in the last decades. They can suppress the formation and/or propagation of cancer cells and are very efficient in cancer therapy.

In the above mentioned group of the steroids, some of the sexual hormones, are in respect to initiation and proliferation of cancer tissue of special interest. They are derived from cholesterol and are transformed by passing intermediate structures to the groups of androgens (governing the male sex characteristics; e.g. testosterone) and estrogens and gestagenes (responsible for female sex; e.g. estradiol, progesterone etc.). The different sexual hormones, androgens and estrogens are generated in both, male and female. However, solely the concentration of given hormone type is the determining factor for the male or female behaviour and sex. The structure formulas of relatively most investigated sexual hormones are shown in Figure11.1.

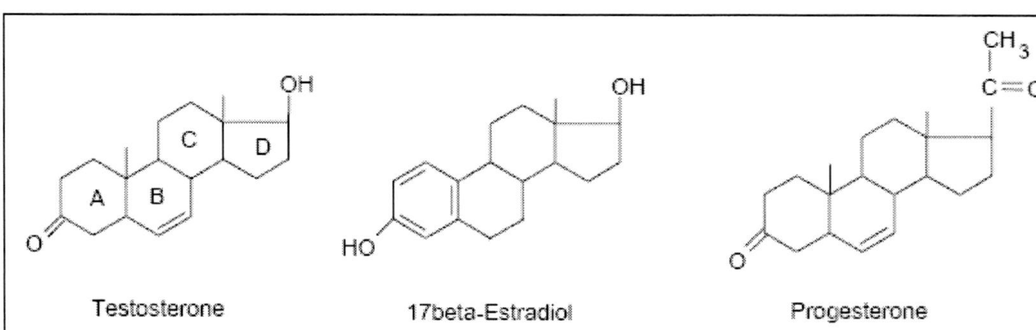

Figure 11.1. Structure formulas of testosterone, 17β-estradiol and progesterone.

An abundant number of papers has been published on the different aspects of sexual hormones, mainly based on studies in vitro /e.g. 2-5/. It was established, that at low concentrations 10^{-8} - 10^{-6} mol/L estradiol stimulates, but at concentrations $\geq 10^{-5}$ mol/L it inhibits the proliferation of cultured endothelial cells of human umbilical cord veins /6/. It was further found, that by implementation of somewhat higher concentrations, A-ring metabolites of 17-β-estradiol (17βE2): 2-hydroxyestrone, 2-hydroxyestradiol, 2-hydroxyestriol, 4-hydroxyestrone and 4-hydroxyestradiol caused a significant inhibition of the cell growth. Hence, 17βE2 hormone and almost all of its A-ring metabolites showed two different effects on cell proliferation: stimulating action at low hormone concentrations ($< 10^{-6}$ mol/L) and inhibition at concentration above 10^{-5} mol/L 17βE2 /7-10/. On the other hand the D-ring of 17βE2 did not show such clear biphasic properties /6/.

For explanation of the carcinogenic effect of estrogens the following mechanisms were postulated /11/: (i) the stimulation of cell proliferation results due to the receptor mediated hormonal activity, (ii) direct genotoxic effects caused through the cytochrome P450 mediated metabolic activation and (iii) by induction of aneuploidy. By testing the natural 17βE2 and its metabolites: 2-hydroxy-, 4-hydroxy- and 16a-hydroxy-estradiol, by inducing neoplastic transformation of human breast epithelial cells in vitro to a degree similar to that generated by the chemical carcinogen benz(a)pyrene, the carcinogenesis of estrogens was demonstrated.

Clinical implications and experimental evidence concerning the initiation of breast cancer by estrogens and some of their metabolites have been comprehensive discussed in recent reviews /12-15/.

11.1. 17β-Estradiol

It should be also mentioned, that 17βE2 hormone regulates several biological processes. It participates not only in the proliferation of normal and breast cancer cells, but also on cell differentiation, reproduction, apoptosis and brain functions /16/. The primary mechanism of 17βE2 biological activity is considered to be initiated by the transcriptional action of the estrogen receptors, ER-α and ER-β, which are members of the large group of highly specialized transcription factors, including the receptors of all steroid hormones /17,18/. Both, ER-α and ER-β receptors, are generally released from inactive complexes, containing heat-shock protein, which can dimerize and bind to a specific DNA-element with response to estrogen and are located in the promotor of target genes /19,20/. In respect to the various cell types and experimental conditions, 17βE2 can effect either decrease or increase of ER-levels. They can be likewise regulated by androgens or progesterone as well as by various growth factors /21,22/. The last ones and 1α,25-dihydroxy vitamin D3 has been found to down-regulate ER-levels /23/.

On the other hand, very recently was established, that 17βE2 and progesterone (PRG) are able to eject or to transfer electrons from their singlet excited state in water-alcohol solvent mixtures to appropriate acceptors /24/. This fact offers a deeper insight and a better understanding of rather complex mechanisms for the carcinogenic behaviour of some 17βE2 metabolites. It was established, that the yield of the generated “solvated electrons” (e_s^-, representing the alkaline form of H-atoms) depends on the molecular hormone structure, substrate concentration, the ratio of water-alcohol solvent mixture as well as on the temperature. Besides, based on the molecular hormone structure the yield of electrons emitted from 17βE2 is two order of magnitude higher that this of PRG. In accordance to earlier findings /25/ the electron emission of 17βE2 takes place from the phenol group (A-ring) of the molecule (see Figure11.1). The A-ring possesses the highest electron density (π-electron structure) resulting into a phenoxyl radical type. This one exists in several mesomeric structures offering a subsequent formation of several metabolites. As already above mentioned the various metabolites on A-ring of 17βE2 own specific biological properties. This fact explains at least partly, the previously discussed carcinogenic behaviour of 17βE2, namely proliferation of normal cells, but also that some of the metabolites may initiate generation of carcinogenic cells.

11.2. Progesterone

On the other side, the electron emission or transfer from PRG to an appropriate acceptor, results into the formation of a progesterone radical cation ($PRG^{\bullet+}$), similar to vitamin E ($vit.E^{\bullet+}$) /26/ and β-carotene radical cations in polar media ($\beta\text{-car}^{\bullet+}$) /27,28/. In general, the radical cations in aqueous media act as strong oxidizing species, since they are leading to formation of OH radicals under regeneration of the substrate, e.g.:

$$\beta\text{-car}^{\bullet+} + H_2O \rightarrow OH + H^+ + \beta\text{-car} \qquad (11.1)$$

or:

$$PRG^{\bullet+} + H_2O \rightarrow OH + H^+ + PRG \qquad (11.2)$$

Subsequently, the OH radicals can attack the components in the given media, according to their reaction rate constants and concentrations. In addition to this the $PRG^{\bullet+}$-transients can principally also regenerate to PRG-hormone by electron transfer from an electron donor, having a suitable redox-potential, e.g. ascorbate anions (AH^-):

$$PRG^{\bullet+} + AH^- \rightarrow PRG + AH^\bullet \qquad (11.3)$$

The resulting vitamin C free radical ($AH^\bullet$) can be involved in other processes or/and undergo disproportion to ascorbic acid (AH_2) and dehydro-ascorbate (DHA), depending on the environment /28/:

$$2\ AH^\bullet \rightarrow AH_2 + DHA \qquad (11.4)$$

In competition to the above processes the $PRG^{\bullet+}$ species can also lead to the formation of metabolites with various properties, as well as such having up or down regulatory effects on the receptor levels in breast cancer cells, as this has been already observed /29/.

11.3. Testosterone

Testosterone (T, 4-androstene-17β-ol-3-on; androgene hormone) is the most investigated male sexual hormone in respect to its relationship to prostate cancer generation and related problems. Earlier studies considered metabolites of testosterone (T) originating from humans, rabbits and rats /30/. In human and male rats kidneys 4-androstene-3,17-dione were detected and to a lesser extent two monohydroxy-monoketo-steroids and dihydroxy-steroids. However, the rabbit kidneys differed from human and rat kidneys by showing a greater rate T-metabolism. Comparing the ability of human prostate cells (LNCaP, DU145, PC3) to metabolize T under living conditions revealed, that their metabolic attitude differed in many respects: (i) rates of precursor degradation, (ii) formation of different products and (iii) extent of conjugate production. Whereas the PC3-cells quickly degraded T an exhibited high formation rate of androstenedione, both DU145 and LNCaP-cells mostly retained high levels of unconverted T. The results demonstrated the rather different action of the various types of cells used as a model for the studies /31/. It also has been established, that 5α-dihydrotestosterone (DHT) is involved in pathogenesis of human prostate cancer /32/. For identification of the metabolites resulting from several cancer cell lines, ^{3}H (tritium) has been used as radio-indicator /33/. It is further noticeable, that androgens play various biological roles. In addition to their action as sexual hormones, they are also involved in cognition and brain aging processes in man /34/.

Finally, it should be noticed, that the mechanisms of the observed effects, particularly those of initiating cancer, are still not satisfactorally lucidated. This is, however, necessary for better understanding the complex biological correlations in order to take required measures for an efficient cancer prevention and therapy. For realization of these objectives it is also needed to clear up the role of the short-lived oxidizing and reducing free radicals, generated in human organisms and their effect on the hormones and in addition to determine the biological action of the resulting final products. Doing so, one can get a so far complete picture of the subject matter and optimize the medical handling of patients.

11. References

[1] Dietrich K., ed., 2001, Encocrinology and Reproduction Medicine, (in German) 4th edition, publ.by Urban and Fischer, Munich and Jena, Germany.

[2] Segaloff A., 1978, Hormons and mammary carcinogenesis, in: "Advances in Research and Treatment of Cancer", pp.1-22, vol.2, ed.McCurie W.L., Plenum, New York, USA.

[3] Garland C.F., Friedlander N.J., et al, 1992, Sex hormones and postmenopausal breast cancer: A prospective study in an adult community, *Amer.J.Epidemol.*135, 1220-1230.

[4] Ioniolo P.G., Levitz M. et al., 1995, A prospective study of endogenous estrogens and breast cancer in postmenopausal women, *J.Nat.Cancer Instr.* 87, 190-197.

[5] Yager J.D., 2000, Endogenous estragens as carcinogens through metabolic activation, *J.Nat.Cancer Inst.Monogr.*27, 67-73.

[6] Lippert C., Seeger H., Mueck A.O. and Lippert T.H., The effects of A-ring and D-ring metabolites of estradiol and the proliferation of vascular endothelial cells, *Life Sciences* 67, 1653-1658.

[7] Mueck A.O., Seeger H. and Lippert T.H., 2002, Estradiol metabolism and malignant disease, Maturitas 43, 1-10.

[8] Lippert C., Seeger H. and Mueck A.O., 2003, The effect of endogenous estradiol metabolites on the proliferation of human breast cancer cells, *Life Sciences* 72, 877-883.

[9] Seeger H., Deuringer F.-U., Wallwiener D. and Mueck A.O., 2004, Breast cancer risk during HRT: Influence of estradiol metabolites on breast cancer and endothelial cell proliferation, *Maturitas* 49, 235-240.

[10] Cupta M., McDouglas A. and Safe S., 1999, Estrogenic and antiestrogenic activities of 16a- and 2-hydroxy metabolites of 17β-estradiol in MCF-7 and T47D-human breast cancer cells, *J.Steroid Biochem.Mol.Biol.67*, 413-419.

[11] Russo J. and Russo I.H., 2006, The role of estrogen in the initiation of breast cancer, *J.Steroid.Biochem.andBiol.*102, 89-96.

[12] Russo J., Lareef M.H., Balogh G., Gao Sh. And Russo I.H., 2003, Estrogen and its metabolites are carcinogenic agents in human breast epithelial cells (review), *J.Steroid.Biochem.andBiol.*87, 1-23.

[13] Pasqualini J.P., 2004, The selective estrogen enzyme modulators in breast cancer: A review, *Biochem.Biophys.Acta* 1654, 123-143.

[14] Yager J.D. and Davidson N.E., 2006, Estrogen Carcinogenesis in breast cancer (Review), *New Engl.J.Med.3*54, 270-282.

[15] Cavalieri D., Chakravarti D.m Guttenplom J et al., 2006, Catecol estrogen quinones as inhibitors of breast and other human cancers: Implication for biomarkers of susceptibility and cancer prevention, *Biochem.Biophys.Acta* 1766, 63-78.

[16] Tsai M.J. and O´Malley B.W., 1994, Molecular mechansim of action of steroid-thyroid receptor superfamily members, *Ann.Rev.Biochem.*63, 451-486.

[17] Zhang D. and Trudeau V.L., 2006, Integration of membrane and nuclear estrogen receptor signaling, *Compt.Biochem.Physiol.A Mol.IntegrPhysiol.*144, 306-315.

[18] Evans R.M., 1988, The steroid and thyroid hormone receptor superfamily, *Science* 240, 889-895.

[19] Boras M., Hardy L., Lempereur F. et al., 1994, Estradiol-induced down regulation of estrogen receptor. Effect of various modulators of protein synthesis and expression, *J.Steroid.Biochem.Mol.Biol.*48, 325-336.

[20] Cowley S.M., Hoare S. et al., 1997, Estrogen receptors alpha and beta heterodimers on DNA, J.Biol.Chem.272, 19858-19862.

[21] El Khissiin A., Cleeren A. et al., 1997, Protein synthesis is not implicated in the ligand-dependent activation of the estrogen receptor in MCF-7 cells, *J.Steroid.Biochem.Mol.Biol.*62, 269-276.

[22] Duffy M.J., 2006, Estrogen receptors: role of breast cancer, *Crit.Rev,Clin.Lab.Sci.* 43, 325-347.

[23] Swami S., Krishnan A.V. and Feldman D., 2000, 1α,25-dihydroxy-vitamin D3 down-regulates estrogen receptor abundance and suppresses estrogen actions in MCF-7 human breast cancer cells, *Cell.Clin.Cancer Res.*6, 3371-3379.

[24] Getoff N, Hartmann J., Huber J.C. and Quint R.M., 2008, Photo-induced electron emission from 17β-Estradiol and Progesterone and possible biological consequences, submitted for publication.

[25] Getoff N., 1989, A review of the relationship between Q(e_{aq}^-) and Q(F) of excited compounds in aqueous solution, *Radiat.Phys.Chem.*34, 711-719.

[26] Getoff N., Platzer I. and Winkelbauer C., 1999, Transients and kooperative action of β-carotene, vitamin E and C in biological systems in vitro under irradiation, *Radiat.Phys,Chem.*55, 699-704.

[27] Getoff N., 2000, Pulse radiolysis studies of β-carotene in oxygenated DMSO solution. Formation of β-carotene radical cation, *Radiat.Res.*154, 692-696.

[28] Kammerer C. and Getoff N., 2004, Synergistic effect of dihydroascorbic acid in mixtures with vitamin E and β-carotene on mitomycin C under irradiation. In Vivo 18, 795-798.

[29] Pawlak K.J. and Wiebe J.P.-, 2007, Regulation of estrogen receptor (ER) levels in MCF-7 cells by progesterone metabolites, *J.Steroid.Biochem.andMol.Biol.*107, 172-179.

[30] Uptila P., Hartiala J. and Nienstedt W., 1980, The metabolism of testosterone by human and rat kidney, *Int.J.Biochem.*12, 345-351.

[31] Castagneta L., Granata O.M., Polito L. et al., 1994, Different conversion metabolitic rates of testosterone are associated to hormone sensitive status and response to human prostate cancer cells, *J.Steroid.Biochem.Mol.Biol.*49, 351-357.

[32] Moneti G., Constantini A., Guana A. et al., 1986, Measurement of testosterone and its 5α-reduced metabolites (DHT and 3α-diol) in human plasma and prostatic tissue by isotopic dilution, *J.Steroid.Biochem.*23, 765-772.

[33] Smith C,M., Ballrad S.A. et al., 1994, Comparison of testosterone metabolism in begin prostate hyperplasia and human prostate cancer cell lines in vitro, *J.Steroid.Biochem.Mol.Biol.*50, 151-159.

[34] Janowsky J.S., 2006, The role of androgens in cognition and brain aging in man, *Neuroscience* 138, 1015-1020.

Chapter 12

Phytohormones

General Remarks

Although nowadays the modern medicine, supported by the strong development of pharmaceutical, electronical industries etc. made an enormous progress, the mother nature is still offering the most intelligent phyto-compounds for combat of cancer and other diseases. The notation phyto-compounds originates from old Greek word "phyton" = plant, which was introduced by Henri Leclere about 100 years ago in medicine and biochemistry. It expresses the biological action of herbs, vegetables and fruits.

The effectiveness of herbal plants was known since 5.000 years and played a basic role in Chinese medicine as well as in Egypt. Some 1.500 years ago the Buddhist monks recommended e.g. garlic as a remedy for many illnesses. The Roman disposed of about 400 plants for production of tea, ointments etc. for prevention and healing of diseases. Some 50 years A.D. the physician of emperor Nero, Dioskurides Pedanios, wrote "De Materia Medica", a pharmacology book summing up the curative action of plants. About the same time Gaius Plinius Secundus comprised the knowledge of the nature sciences in 37 volumes "Naturalis Historia", where the plants and their implementation in the medicine is content in 8 volumes. Later on, in the middle ages the monks in various monasteries continued the successfully use of herbs and vegetables for the prevention and curing of sickness. However, with the development of synthetic drugs, the knowledge of the curative action of plants was nearly lost and forgotten. At first with ending of the 19th and beginning of the 20th century the interest to the biological action of herbs and their use in the medicine arose again. Nowadays the use of phyto-compounds for prevention purposes as well as the modern phyto-therapy is so far developed, that it strongly differs from the traditional medicine sciences. The phyto-drugs are now available in permanent high quality.

Supplementary might be mentioned, that the plants, vegetables and fruits are consisting mainly of water. The remaining organic compounds comprises of about 95% carbohydrates, fats, vitamins, proteins, and minerals. The vestige of 5% represents biological active polyphenols and phenolic acids (coffeic acid, ferula acids, etc.), flavonoids (e.g. resveratrol, catechin), isoflavones (phytohormones), carotinoids (α-, β-carotenes, lycopin, lutein etc.), phytosterines (genistein, daidzen, etc.) and saponins (ginseng etc.) All these substances offer the plants taste, aroma and protection against pests, pathogenic agents, protection against UVsunlight, heat and coldness. The phyto-compounds consumed as nutrients can also protect human organism against cancer, cardio-vascular, infections and other diseases.

The coffee and ferula acids are the most common polyphenols in plants, fruits and vegetables and are chemically bonded on sugars, flavonoids and plant-sterins. Since plant extracts are of importance for human nutrition, their biochemical activity has been widely investigated. Studies showed, that more than 40% of the investigated flavonoids are present in the gastrointestinal tract of the organism.

The group of flavonoids and anthrocyanes grasps about 6.500 compounds, which are basically consisting of three carbon-rings and are also mainly chemically bonded to sugars and phenolic acids. The most of the flavonoids are yellow coloured (lat. flavus = yellow), whereas the anthocyanes are responsible, as mentioned above for the red, blue and violet colours of the flowers etc.

The polyphenols have many-folded biological effects and can influence the human health in different ways including the prevention of cancer. Similar to their action in plants, they can protect humans from various illnesses and extend various curative effects. They can also act as rather potent biochemical antioxidants scavenging oxidizing free radicals (OH, $O_2^{\bullet-}$, etc.), especially in the digestive tract in the organism and prevent from deleterious consequences, such as cancer and geriatric complaints.

In the frame of exhaustive pulse radiolysis experiments the spectral and kinetic acid-base and redox-properties of the resulting phenoxyl radicals of selected flavonoides were investigated /1/. The dissociation constants (pK_1, pK_2 and pK_3) of flavonones, flavones and phenols, as well as electron-transfer reactions of $O_2^{\bullet-}$ radical anions by flavonoids and phenols were determined.

A consecutive two-electron oxidation process has been suggested for the reaction of peroxyl radical ($RO_2^{\bullet}$) with 3´,4´- or 2´,5´-dihydroxyflavonols under the formation of the corresponding quinines (see eq.12.1). The first oxidation step leads to the formation of flavonoid phenoxyl radical, which subsequently react with a second $RO_2^{\bullet}$ species to result into the corresponding quinines. Thereby both reaction steps take place predominantly on the B-ring of the compound (eq.12.1):

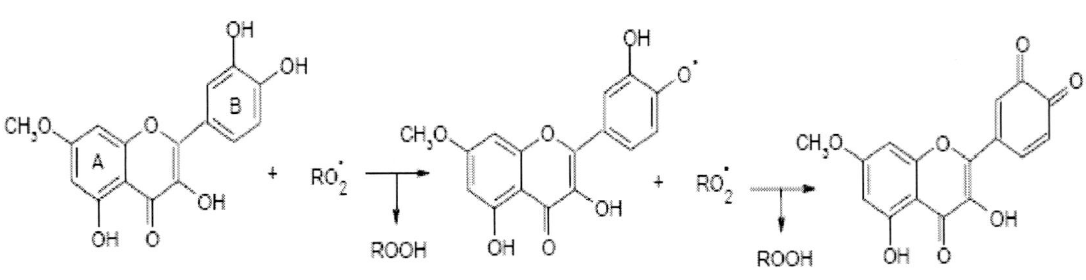

Eq. 12.1. Selective attack of organic peroxyl radicals on the B-ring of dihydroxyflavonoides.

As already mentioned the polyphenols contained in vegetables, fruits, wines, spices and herbal medicines exert numerous of beneficial antioxidant, anticancer and antiflamatory properties. It is also found that dietary polyphenols were metabolized by peroxidase forming phenoxyl radicals (see eq. 12.1), which can cooxidase GSH and NADH /2/. This is accompanied in some cases by extensive oxygen uptake. Similar antioxidant effects were observed by use of various dietary flavonoids /3/. On the other hand it was reported that peroxynitrite and NO^- can initiate an ortho-trihydroxyl group, acting as pro-oxidant /4/.

It is also to be mentioned, that aqueous phenol and related compounds can eject or transfer electron from their singlet excited states /5/. Hence, polyphenols are acting as very potent electron donors, resulting into phenoxyl radical, which has several mesomeric forms (eqs. 12.2 and 12.3). Each of them can subsequently lead to the formation of a specific product.

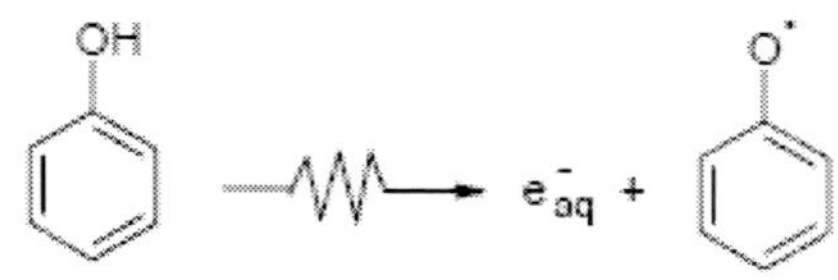

(12.2)

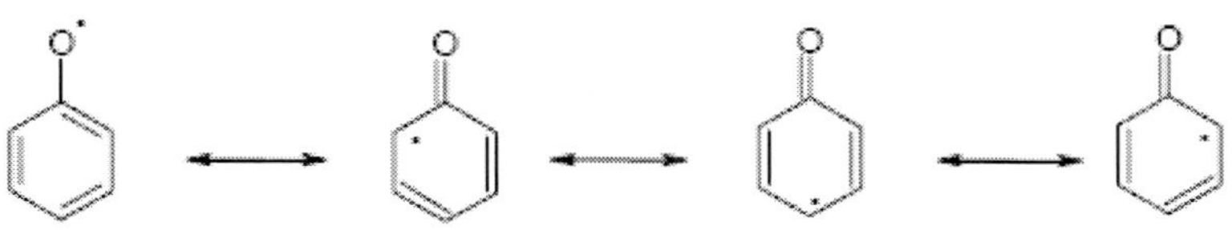

(12.3)

Some representative phyto-compounds having antitumor properties are discussed in some detail.

12.1. Resveratrol

Resveratrol (trans-3,4′,5-trihydoxystilbene, phytoalexin, trans-resveratrol, RES) is found in grapes, red wine, cranberries, peanuts, red clover and in variety of plants and fruits. It is a naturally occurring antibiotic, used as an active ingredient in Asian Folk medicine, because of its various antipathogenic properties. It has been found to account at least in part for the so-called “French-paradox”, i.e. the fact that incidence of myocardial infraction in Southern France is about 40% lower than in the rest of Europe, despite the population′s high fat diet and cigarette comsume. Based on this fact and on its antitumor property RES become an interesting research object. This resulted in a very large number of publications, reporting on the antioxidant, peroxidant as well as antitumor properties of RES /e.g. 6-9/. The fact concerning the various biological features of RES has been excellently reviewed by Aggarwal et al. /10/.

Some very recent data demonstrating the broad biological action of RES are briefly discussed. First, for convenience the structure formula of RES is given in Figure 12.1. The three hydroxyl groups of RES molecule account for its electron-donor ability, whereas the π-electron structure of the phenolic and resorcinol rings for its high reactivity with free radicals.

Based on the fact, that human organism generates oxidizing (OH, $O_2^{\bullet-}$ etc.) and reducing free radicals (e_{aq}^-, $R^\bullet$ etc.), which are involved in various important biological functions, their effect on RES was investigated in vitro. As a model for living systems MCF-7 cancer cells were investigated under various experimental conditions /11/. Thereby γ-ray were used for the generation of the corresponding free radicals.

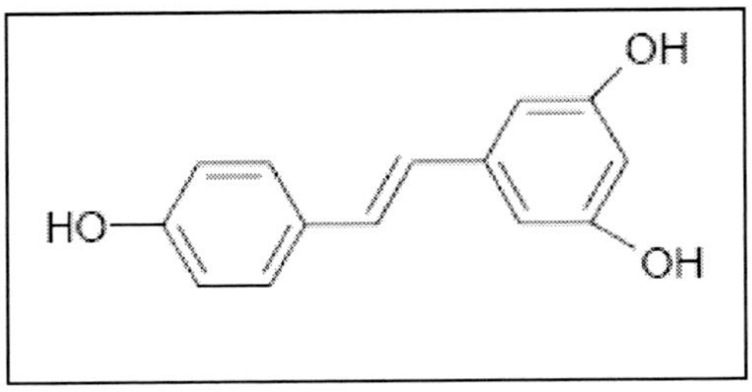

Figure 12.1. Structure formula of resveratrol.

Some data derived from survival curves obtained at pH=7.4 in the presence and absence of air and in aqueous media saturated with N_2O (conversion of e_{aq}^- into OH radicals) are presented in Table 12.1. Additionally, experiments containing 1 mmol formate (transforming of OH and H radicals into e_{aq}^- in airfree environment) were also reported. The antitumor action of RES and mitomycin C (MMC) as well as mixtures of both are also compared /11/. The reactions 12.4 to 12.7 visualize the conversion of OH and H radicals into e_{aq}^-.

$$OH + HCOO^- \rightarrow H_2O + {}^{\bullet}COO^- \quad (k = 2.7 \times 10^9\ L.mol^{-1}.s^{-1}) \qquad (12.4)$$

$$H + HCOO^- \rightarrow H_2 + {}^{\bullet}COO^- \quad (k = 2.5 \times 10^8\ L.mol^{-1}.s^{-1}) \qquad (12.5)$$

$$COO^- + MMC \rightarrow CO_2 + MMC^{\bullet -} \quad \text{(MMC-semiquinone)} \qquad (12.6)$$

$$e_{aq}^- + MMC \rightarrow MMC^{\bullet -} \quad (k = 2.2 \times 10^{10}\ L.mol^{-1}.s^{-1}) \qquad (12.7)$$

$MMC^{\bullet -}$ species are the acting form of MMC /12 and refs. therein/. It has been established, that the OH-adducts and the peroxyl-radicals of MMC show a strong cytostatic action /13/ (see also chapter 4.2.).

Table 12.1. $\Delta N/N_0$-ratio *) of survival MCF-7 cancer cells in various media, after treatment with γ-ray (5 Gy absorbed radiation dose)

System	$\Delta N/N_0$-ratios in different media: A. Air 46% OH, 54% $O_2^{\bullet -}$	B. N_2O 90% OH, 10% H	C. Airfree **) 100% e_{aq}^-
2 μmol RES	0.120	0.125	0.20
50 μmol RES	0.03	- 0.120	0.08
1 μmol MMC	0.28	0.270	-0.22
2 μmol RES + 1 μmol MMC	0.68	0.110	-0.05
50 μmol RES + 1 μmol MMC	0.32	-0.070	-0.12

*) $\Delta N/N_0 = N/N_0(\text{system}) - N/N_0(\text{buffer})$, where N_0 = number of cells before and N = number of cells after treatment with 5 Gy γ-ray. The positive data indicate the radical scavenging ability of the system, whereas the negative ones show the antitumor effect.

**) In the presence of 1 mmol formate (see reactions: 12.4 to 12.7)

The $\Delta N/N_0$-data observed for 2 μmol RES in all media that RES is an efficient radical scavenger, favouring the proliferation of the cancer cells. This effect is, however, strongly reduced in media (A) by using 50 μmol RES. In media (B) it shows even a very strong cytostatic action ($\Delta N/N_0$ = - 0.120). By implementation of formate (column C) for transformation of OH and H into e_{aq}^- (creation of a strong reducing environment), both RES concentration (2 and 50 μmol) display a protection against free radicals. However, using 50 μmol RES in airfree media the antitumor effect of RES (similar as in column A) is beginning to play a role. On the other hand the implementation of 1 μmol MMC in combination with RES in oxidizing media (column A and B) leads to a protection of the cancer cells (the system acts as a potent radical scavenger). But, in the presence of formate (action of e_{aq}^- only) a strong cytostatic behaviour for both mixtures is observed. This effect increases essentially with the enhancement of the RES concentration, demonstrating its electron donor ability thus raising the $MMC^{\bullet-}$ formation. Similar effect, but much weaker expressed, is registered for the mixture of 1 μmol MMC and 50 μmol RES in media (B), where 10% H atoms are also acting.

Summing up it can be stated, that RES exhibits bifunctional properties: it acts as a potent radical scavenger, as well as a very efficient antitumor substance, attributed to its ability to effect or/and transfer electrons, depending on the redox-potential of the reaction partner.

Final Products of Resveratrol. The reaction of free radicals in organism with pharmaceutics, phyto-compounds, nutrients, etc. in organism is leading to the formation of numerous final products. These can have a positive biological effect or can be subsequently involved in various processes, causing undesired biological actions and initiate sicknesses. Therefore, it is of advantage to have an indication about the products resulting from RES as a sequence of such reactions. Studies in this respect have been performed in aqueous solutions, using γ-ray to generate the desired primary free radicals involved in the RES degradation, and the resulting final products /14/. It has been established that mainly the oxidizing radicals (OH, $O_2^{\bullet-}$) are leading to the formation of a mixture of aldehydes, carboxylic acids etc. in addition to 3,5-dihydroxy-benzoic acid as a main product. Thereby at an absorbed radiation dose of 500 Gy, corresponding to about 19 μmols free radicals, the product formation is proportional to the radical concentration.

As a conclusion it can be stated that RES is a compound with unique biological properties. In addition to its strong antitumor effect, it is a very efficient radical scavenger, particularly of OH and peroxyl radicals. The products resulting by the oxidative RES-degradation, particularly aldehydes, when formed in somewhat higher concentration, are injurious to health.

12.2. Genistein

Genistein (4',5,7-trihydroxyisoflavone) is a phyto-estrogen, belonging to the group of isoflavonoids. It is contained in relatively high concentration in soybeans (in addition to genistin and daidzin) as well as in red clover and many other plants ect. /15,16/. (see Figure 10.2). Genistein (GEN) is consumed as food and is proved in serum of humans and animals. Similar to other estrogen-hormons it exhibits the same biological properties, however, in weaker form. It has been found that GEN is involved in several processes, e.g. reduction of

DNA oxidative damage and lipide peroxidation /17/, regulation of HMG-CoA-reductase in MCF-7 human breast cancer cells /18/, increase of the radiation effect in cervical cancer cells /19/, holding up of invasive potential of human hepato cellular carcinoma by altering cell cycle /20/, the effect of the synthetic isoflavone, phenosodiol, in the course of ovarian and other kinds of human cancer /21/. The anticancer properties of soya isoflavones has been also exhaustively discussed in a review paper /22/. The various action of GEN can be conducted back to its very high reactivity to OH-radicals, reaction rate constant, $k = 2.3 \times 10^{10}$ $L.mol^{-1}.s^{-1}$ at pH = 8.3 /23/ and to that of the "solvated electrons" (e_{aq}^-), $k = 6.2 \times 10^9$ $L.mol^{-1}.s^{-1}$ in neutral aqueous media /24/.

As already mentioned in previous chapters, the human organism is generating oxidising (OH, $O_2^{\bullet -}$ etc.) as well as reducing free radicals (e_{aq}^-, H, etc.), which are indispensable for the unobjectionable function of numerous biological processes. For example, the oxidative free radicals are involved in reactions with nutrients in respect to their decomposition. On the other hand for the right function, particulary of the nervous system, communication between cells etc., the "solvated electrons" (e_{aq}^-) as well as electron transfer processes are responsible. Naturally, consumed pharmaceutica and related substances are also involved in reactions with free radicals.

Based on these facts, studies concerning the processes initiated by free radicals attack on GEN has been very recently reported /25/. By implementation of MCF-7 human breast cancer cells as a model, the biological properties of GEN after treatment with γ-ray (absorbed dose 5 Gy) in various media were investigated. Under these experimental conditions different types of free radicals are operating. Based on the water radiolysis data (see chapter 2, Table 2.1), where the yields of primary radicals generated by a dose of 1 Gy is 6.344×10^{-7} mol/L (e_{aq}^- + H + OH), the corresponding percentages were calculated. The observed results under reported experimental conditions are presented in Figure 12.3, where the content of each system is shown as individual column (see also /25/). For comparison two GEN-concentrations as well as mitomycin C (MMC) and mixture of GEN and MMC were also studied.

In aqueous media saturated with air, only oxidizing free radicals are operating (see Figure 12.3). In view of columns (A) to (E) it is evident, that the N/N_0-values are decreasing, indicating the increase of the antitumor effect of the corresponding system. With increasing the GEN-concentration (column B and C, Figure 12.3) also its antitumor effect rises slowly, but is not proptortional to the GEN-concentration and is still lower than that of MMC (column D).

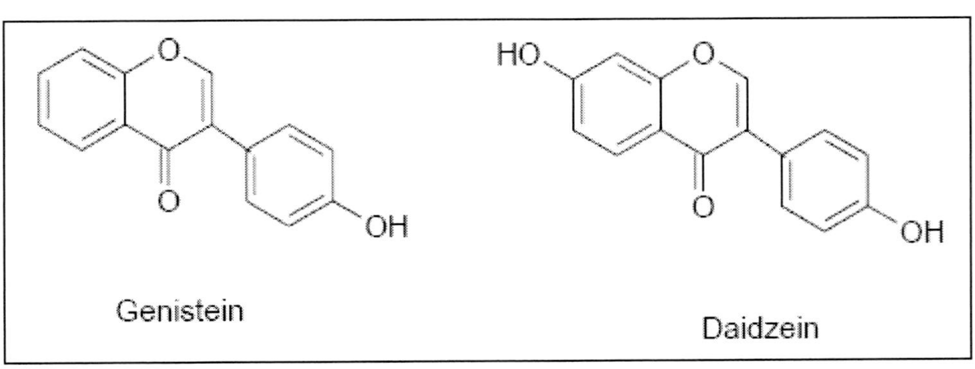

Fig.12.2. Structure of genistein and daidzein.

It is, however, interesting, that MMC efficiency is increased in the presence of GEN (column E). This indicates a synergistic effect of GEN enhancing the MMC activity.

In the case of the results obtained in media saturated with N_2O (Figure12.3), where 10% H and 90% OH radicals are operating, a rather similar situation is principally observed, but the synergistic effect of GEN is somewhat stronger pronounced (compare column D and E). The synergistic effect of GEN is particulary marked in media saturated with Argon, where the reducing radicals predominate, column C, D and E have the lowest N/N_0-values. The synergistic effect of GEN, represented by column E shows $N/N_0 = 0.25$ compared to those in aerated media ($N/N_0 = 0.48$) and N_2O containing ones ($N/N_0 = 0.38$). This indicates the highest antitumor effect in airfree media.

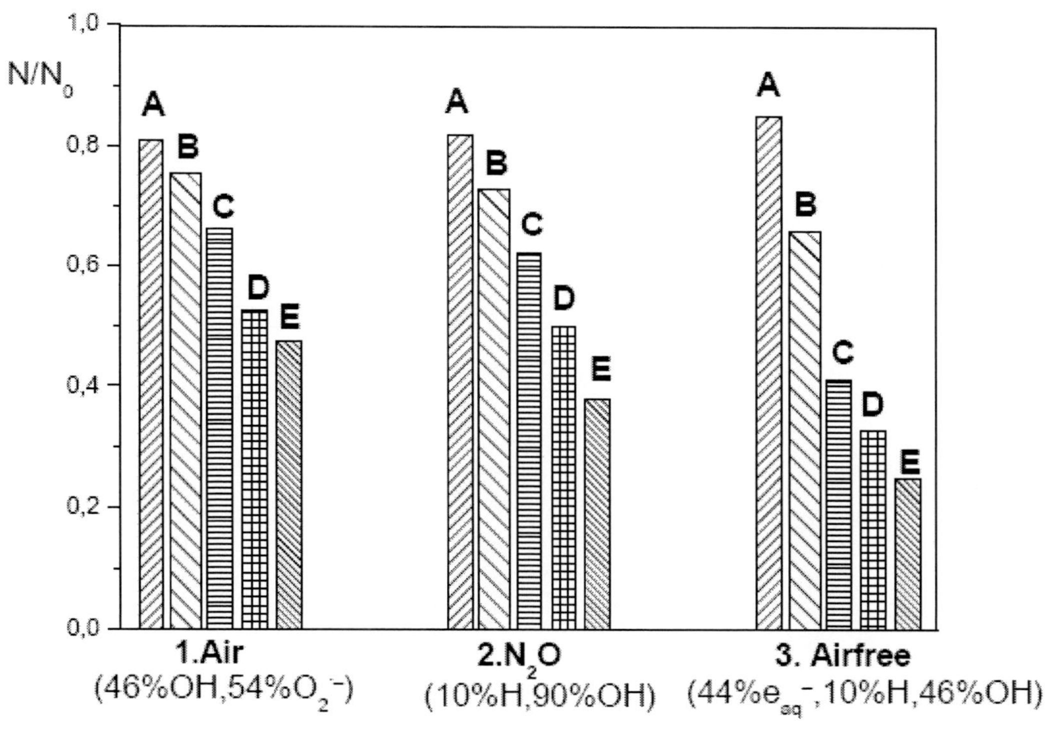

Figure 12.3. N/N_0-survival ratio of MCF-7 cancer cells after treatment with γ-ray (5 Gy absorbed dose) in aqueous media (pH = 7.4): (1) aerated, (2) saturated with N_2O and (3) saturated with argon. The solution content in individual columns is: (A) buffer, (B) 5 μmol GEN, (C) 40 μmol GEN, (D) 2.5 μmol MMC, (E) 2.5 μmol MMC + 40 μmol GEN; where: N_0 = number of cells before radiation treatment, N = after that. Remark: The lower the N/N0-ratio of a given system, the higher is its anticancer effect.

Based on the reported results the following conclusion has been made: (1) GEN acts as an efficient radical scavenger (see also the reaction rate constant for e_{aq}^- and OH radicals. (2) GEN shows antitumor property, which is rising with increase of its concentration. (3) The antitumor effect of GEN is weaker than that of MMC, but this could be compensated by higher GEN-concentrations. (4) It appears, that GEN is an efficient electron donor. This explains its synergistic effect to MMC, particulary in airfree media, since it leads to the formation of a higher $MMC^{\bullet -}$ (semiquinone) concentration. As it has been shown earlier (see chapter 4.2.) the highest action of MMC is its semiquinone form, although the other MMC-transients such as OH-adducts (MMC.OH), peroxyl-radicals ($MMC.O_2^{\bullet}$) and radical cation ($MMC^{\bullet +}$) likewise have a cytostatica effect feature, but with lower efficiency.

It is of interest to be mentioned, that the attack of free racials on genistein in aerated neutral aqueous media is leading to the formation of some final products /26/. Under given circumstances they can play a biological role (side effects). In addition to qercetin, appearing as a main product, also a mixture of aldehydes, carboxylic acids and a number of unidentified substances with small yields were detected by HPLC-analysis.

12.3. Daidzein

Daidzein (7-hydroxy-3-(hydroxyphenyl)-4H-1-benzopyran-4-one; 4'-7-dihydroxy-isoflavone) is naturally found, like genistein, as glycoside in soybeans and is the second most abudant isoflavone. It is also classified as a phytoestrogen, since it possesses estrogen-like biological effect, but it shows also anti-estrogenic action. Daidzein is the aglycone of daidzin, likewise naturally occuring as glycoside daidzin. Both, daidzein and daidzin are also found in Radix puerariae /27/. It is also used as a herbrae drug for centuries in the traditional Chinese medicine for treatment of several disorders /28/ as well as for "anti-drunkness" /29, 30/. Daidzein has the lowest estrogenic effect of the soy-isoflavones. It is explected, that it can have also some anticancer properties /31/.

12. References

[1] Jovanovic S.V., Steenken S., Tosic M., Marjanovic B.and Simic M.G., 1994, Flavonoids as antioxidants, *J.Am.Chem.Soc.*116, 4846-4851.

[2] Galati G., Sabzevari O., Wilson J.X. and O´Brien P.J., 2002, Prooxidant activity and cellular effects of the phenoxyl radicals of dietary flavonoids and other polyphenols, *Toxicology* 177, 91-104.

[3] Cai Q., Rahn O.R. and Zhang R., 1997, Dietary flavonoids, quercetin, luteolin and genistein reduce oxidative DNA damage and lipid peroxidation and quench free radicals, *Cancer Letters* 119, 99-107.

[4] Ohshima H., Yoshic Y., Auriol S. and Gilibert I., 1998, Antioxidant and pro-oxidant actions of flavonoids: Effects on DNA damage induced by nitric oxide, peroxynitrite and nitroxyl anion, *Free Rad.Biology and Med.*25, 1057-1065.

[5] Getoff N., 1989, A review of the relationship between $Q(e_{aq}^-)$ and Q(F) of excited compounds in aqueous solution, Radiat.Phys.Chem.34, 711-719.

[6] Fuggetta M.P., D'Atri S., Lanzilli G., Tricarico M., Cannavo E., Zambruno G., Falchetti R. and Ravagnan G., 2004, In vitro antitumor activity of resveratrol in human melanoma cells sensitive or resistent to temozolomode, *Melanoma Res.*14, 189-196.

[7] Levi F., Pasche C., Lucchini F., Guidoni R., Ferrarono M. and LaVechia C., 2005, Resveratrol and breast cancer risk, *Eur.J.Cancer Prev.*14, 139-142.

[8] Marier J.F., Chen K., Prince P., Scott G., DelCastillo J.R. and Vachon P., 2005, Production of ex vivo lipopolisaccharide-induced tumor necrosis factor alpha,

interleukin-1-beta and interleukin-6 is suppressed by trans-resveratrol in a concentration depended manner, *Can.J.Vet.Res.*69, 151-154.

[9] Murias M., Jaeger W., Handler N., Erker T., Horvath Z., Szekeres T., Nohl H. and Gille L., 2005, Antioxidant and cytotoxic activity of hydroxylated resveratrol analogues: structure-activity relationship, *Biochem.Pharmacol.*69, 903-912.

[10] Aggarwal B.B., Bhardwaj A., Aggarwal R.S., Seeram N.P., Shissshodia S. and Takada Y., 2004, Role of resvertrol in prevention and therapy of cancer preclinical and clinical studies, *Anticancer Res.*24, 2783-2840.

[11] Bader Y. and Getoff N., 2006, Effect of resveratrol and mixtures of resveratrol and mitomycin C on cancer cells under irradiation, *Anticancer Res.*26, 4403-4408.

[12] Getoff N., 2001, Cytostatic efficiency enhancement by vitamins C, E, and β-carotene under irradiation. State of the art, *Radiat.Phys.Chem.*60, 351-358.

[13] Getoff N., Solar S. and Quint R.M., 1997, One-electron oxidation of mitomycin C and its corresponding peroxyl-radical. A steady-state and pulse radiolysis sturdy, *Radiat.Phys.Chem.*50, 575-583.

[14] Bader Y., Quint R.M. and Getoff N., 2007, Resveratrol products resulting by free radicals attack, Radiat.Phys.Chem., *in print.*

[15] Dietrich K. (ed.), 2001, Endokrinology and Reproduction Medicine I. (in German), Publ.Comp.UrbanandFischer, Munich and Jena.

[16] Dixon R.A. nd Ferreira D., 2002, Molecules of interest. Genistein, Phytochemistry 60, 205-211.

[17] Cai Q., Rahn O.R. and Zang R., 1997, Dietary flavonoids, quercetin, luteolin and genistein reduce oxidative DNA damage nad lipide peroxidation and qench free radicals, *Cancer Letters* 119, 99-107.

[18] Duncan R.E., El-Sohemy A. and Archer M.C., 2005, Regulation of HMG-CoA reductase in MCF-7 cells by genistein, EPA and DHA alone and in combination with mevastin, *Cancer Letters* 224, 221-228.

[19] Yashar G.M., Spanos W.J. et al., 2005, Potentiation of radiation effect with genistein in cervical cancer ceklls, *Gynecol.Oncology* 99, 199-205.

[20] Gu Y., Zhe C.F. et al., 2005, Genistein inhibits invasive potential of human hepatocellular carcinoma by altering cell cycle apoptosis and angiogenesis, *World J. Gastroenterol.* 11, 6512-6517.

[21] Morre D.J., Chuch P.-J., et al., 2007, Ecto-nox target for the anticancer isoflavone phenoxodiol, *Oncology Res.*16, 299-312.

[22] Ravindram M.H., Muthugounder N. et al., 2004, Anticancer therapoitic potenital of soy isoflavone, genistein. Review, *Adv.Exp.Med.Biol.*546, 121-165.

[23] Zielonka J., Gebicki J. and Grynkiewicz G., 2003, Radical scanvenging properties of genistein, *Free Radical Biology and Medicine* 35, 958-965.

[24] Cai Z., Ku X. and Katsumura Y., 1999, Interaction of hydrated electron with dietary flavonoids and phenolic acids. Rate constants and transient spectra studied by pulse radiolysis, *Free Radical Biol.andMed.*27, 822-829.

[25] Hartmann J. and Getoff N., 2008, Effect of free radicals on the biological action of genistein studied in vitro. Synergism to mitomycin C, Anticancer Res., *submitted for publication..*

[26] Hartmann J., Quint R.M. and Getoff N., 2007, Products resulting by free radical attack on aqueous genistein, *Radiat.Phys.Chem., in print,*

[27] Keung W.-M-, Lazo O., et al., 1996, Potentiation of the bioavailability of daidzin by an extract of Radix puerariae, *Proc.Natl.Acad.Sci. USA* 93, 4284-4288.

[28] Keung W.-M. and Vallee B.L., 1998, Daidzin and its antidipsotropic analogs inhibit serotonin and dopamine metabolism in isolated mitochondria, *Proc.Natl.Acad.Sci. USA* 95, 2198-2203.

[29] Keung W.-M., Vallee B.L., 1993, Daidzin and daidzein suppress free-choice ethanol intake by Syrian Golden hamsters, *Proc.Natl.Acad.Sci. USA* 90, 1008-1012.

[30] Keung W.-M., Kazo O. and Vallee B.L., 1995, Daidzin suppresses ethanol consumption by Syrian Golden Hamsters without blocking acet-aldehyde metabolism, *Proc.Natl.Acad.Sci. USA* 92, 8990-8993.

[31] Sugiomoto E. and Yamaguchi M., 2000, Stimulatory effect of daidzein in osteoblastic MC3T3-E1 cells, *Biochem.Pharmacol.*59, 471-475.

Chapter 13

Nutrition and Cancer

It is well known, that the prevention and in some cases even the therapy of cancer can be positively influenced by dietary modification. The nutrition is presently a rather modern area of clinical and epidemiological research. In the frame of studies by EPIC (European Prospective Investigation into Cancer and Nutrition), where 23 centers from 10 countries are participating, the following data have been established /1/.

- The consumption of fruits is negatively associated with cancer of the lung, but probably not with prostate and breast cancer.
- Taking vegetables, mainly onion and garlic, reduces the risk of intestinal stomach cancer, but is probably not associated with cancer of the lung, prostate and breast.
- Fish consumption is negative associated with colorectal cancer risk, however, intake of red and processed meat is positively associated with colorectal cancer and with non-cardia stomach cancer in those infected by Heliobacter pylori.
- Finally, high alcohol consumption increases the risk of breast cancer.

These results from the EPIC-study on some food groups provide a scientific knowledge for appropriate public strategies for reducing the global cancer burden.

Simultaneously with the evidence about the dietary components determining cancer risk and tumor behaviour, also papers showing discrepancies in this respect have been published /2/. It appears that many factors, e.g. genetic polymorphisms, can influence metabolism or site of action, variation of DNA-methylation pattern etc., can effect the biological response to food components. Therefore, evaluating the significance of the interrelationship among bioactive food components with nutritional epigenomics is necessary in order to get a more clear picture about the relation of nutrition and cancer /3/.

Aside from these findings, very intense studies concerning the effect of various kinds of food on carcinogenesis were performed recently. Conducted examination on the relationship between intake of fruit, vegetables as well as soy food appearance of breast cancer in Korean women was found /4/: (1) No association between the intake of total fruits, vegetables or soy food and breast cancer risk was found. (2) With high tomato intake a reduced cancer risk was observed; (3) Increased consumption of grapes was linked to a rather significant protective effect against risk of breast cancer and, (4) an increased intake of cooked yellow and black soy beans lead to reduced breast cancer. The major glycolipids fraction contained in spinach inhibited proliferation of human cervix carcinoma (HeLa) cells /5/. Zapotin (5,6,2',6'-tetramethoxyflavone) found in the tropical fruit zapote blanco (casimiroa edulis) showed a marked suppression of cell proliferation (HT-29) /6/. The consumption of coffee and tea has been also investigated in respect to cancer. Studies showed, that increased consumption of coffee might be positively associated with ovarian cancer risk. However, the epidemiologic evidence regarding tea intake and ovarian cancer is inconsistent /7/. This was reported as a result of follow-up 264 incident ovarian cancer cases during a period of more than 16 years. These findings were confirmed by further studies in this respect /8, 9/.

An abundant literature is concerned with the postitive dietary effects of soy products /10, 11/. In this respect the special role of flavonoids (genistein, biochanin A) on gene expression and their metabolism in human mammary cells was investigated /12/. Their preventive properties towards prostate cancer /13-15/, colon cancer /16/ as well as of breast cancer were reported /17/. A systematic literature search of papers published in any language upto 2006 has been conducted to identify the reports concerning the intake of fruits and vegetables in relation to cancer /18/. The search suggested a modest inverse association with vegetable consumption, particularly for cruciferons vegetables. No studies were found evaluating the intake of fruits and vegetables separately in order to establish their individual biological consequences.

Investigations concerning antioxidant phytocompounds in fresh samples of edible maturity stage in different cruciferous vegetables, showed that the highest content was established in broccoli. In 100 g broccoli were found: 52.9 mg vitamin C, 0.81 mg β-carotene, 0.68 mg lutein, 0.47 mg DL-α-tocopherol and 63.4 mg phenol. The results indicate that the cruciferous vegetables are good source of abundant antioxidants. Summing up it is noticed that nowdays the determining role of nutrition in respect to cancer is well established and a modern branch of medicine is involved in this domain.

Sterilization and Preservation of Food

Just for completeness of the subject matter it is briefly mentioned that the very rapid increase of the world population, particularly in the developing countries, bring forth enormous nutrition problems.

In order to extend the life-time of storage of agricultural products as well as fish, meat, poultery etc. and on the other hand to reduce the risk for inadvertently transporting quarantine pests and transfer of sicknesses to countries or regions, where they do not occure, sanitary treatments (fumigation, heat, cold or radiation) were suggested. Among these methods, irradiation under strongly determined conditions is recognized as a versatile treatment of food. It offers a broad spectrum of activity and minimum adverse effects on the quality of most commodities /20/.

13. References

[1] Gonzales C.A. and Riboli E., 2006, Diet and cancer prevention: where we are, where we are going, *Nutr.Cancer* 56, 225-231.

[2] Milner J.A., 2006, Diet and cancer: facts and controversies, Nutr.Cancer 56, 216-224.

[3] Chamras H., Barsky S.H., Ardashian A. et al., 2005, Novel interactions of vitamin E and Estrogen in breast cancer, *Nutr.Cancer* 52, 43-48.

[4] Mh Do, Lee S.S., Jung P.J. and Lee Mh., 2007, Intake of fruits, vegetables and soy foods in relation to breast cancer risk in Korean women. A case-control study, *Nutr.Cancer* 57, 20-27.

[5] Maeda N., Kokai Y., Ohtan S., et al., 2007, Antitumor effects of the glycolipids fraction from spinach which inhibited DNA polymerase activity, *Nutr.Cancer* 37, 216-223.

[6] /6/ Murillo G., Hirschelman W.H., Ito A. et al., 2007, Zapotin, a phytochemical present in a Mexican fruit, prevents colon carcinogenesis, *Nutr.Cancer* 57, 28-37.

[7] Silvera S.A., Jain M. et al., 2007, Intake of coffee and tea and risk of ovarian cancer : A prospective cohort study, *Nutr.Cancer* 58, 22-27.

[8] /8/ Mandal D., Bhattacharyya S. et al., 2007, Black tea-induced decrease in IL-10 adn TGF-beta of tumor cell promotes Th1/Te1 response in tumor bearer, *Nutr.Cancer* 58, 213-221.

[9] Hao X., Sun Y., Yang C.S. et al., 2007, Inhibition of intestinal tumorigenesis in Ape(min/+)mice by green tea polyphenols (polyphenon E) and individual catechins, *Nutr.Cancer* 59, 62-69.

[10] Ursin G., Sun C.L., Koh W.P. et al., 2006, Associates between soy diet, reproductive factors and mammography densitiy in Singapore Chinese women, *Nutr.Canc*er 56, 128-135.

[11] Takata Y., Maskarinec G., et al., 2006, Serum insulin-like growth factor-I levels among women in Hawaii and Japan with different levels of tofu intake, *Nutr.Cancer* 56, 136-142.

[12] Moon Y.J., Brazean D.A. and Morris M.E., 2007, Effect of flavonoids, genestein and biochanin A on gene expression and their metabolism in human mammary, *Nutr.Cancer* 57, 48-58.

[13] DeWell A., Weidner G., Summer M.D. et al., 2007, Relationship of dietary protein and soy isoflavones to serum IGF-1 and IGF binding proteins in the prostate cancer lifestyle trial, *Nutr.Cancer* 58, 35-42.

[14] McCormick D.L., Johnson W.D., Bosland M.C. et al., 2007, Chemoprevention of rat prostata carcinogenesis by soy isoflavones and by Bowman-Birk inhibitor, *Nutr.Cancer* 57, 184-193.

[15] Kumar N.B., Krischer J.P., Allen K. et al., 2007, Safety of purified isoflavones in man with clinically localized prostata cancer, *Nutr.Cancer* 59, 169-175.

[16] Oba S., Nagata C., Shimizu N. et al., 2007, Soy product consumption and the risk of colon cancer: A preventive study in Kakayama, Japan, *Nutr.Cancer* 57, 151-157.

[17] Toneti D.A., Zhang Y., Zhao H. et al., 2007, The effect of the phytoestrogenes genistein, daidzein and equol on the growth of tamoxifen-restistant T47D/PKC alpha, *Nutr.Cancer* 58, 222-229.

[18] Banera E.V., Kushi L.H., Moore D.F. et al., 2007, Fruits and vegetables and endometrial cancer risk: A systematic literature review and meta-analysis, *Nutr.Cancer* 58, 6-21.

[19] Biesalski H.-K., Fuerst P., Kasper H., et al., eds., 2004, Nutrition Medicine (in German), Georg Thieme Publ.House, Stuttgart and New York.

[20] Irradiation as a phytosanitary treatment of food and agricultural commodities, IAEA-TECDOC-1427, Nov.2004, IAEA, Vienna, Austria.

Chapter 14

Environmental Factors as Cancer Inititators

As a consequence of the rapid development of various industries and the very strong growth of the world population a rather heavy overloading of water resources and air is observed. By combustion of fossil fuels (coal, oil, natural gas) a number of polycyclic aromatid hydrocarbons (PAH's) are generated, which are very toxic and carcinogenic /1/. In addition to the industries also large power stations are emitting enormous quantities of CO_2 and PAH's. To that the exhaust gasses of motor-cars, particulary by heavy traffic in the rush hours in big citys, strongly contribute to the pollution of air and water resources. The toxicity and carcinogenity of PAH's compounds roughly increases with the enhancement of their molecular weight, e.g. the maximum permissible concentration of fluorene is 0.002, fluoranthene 0.001 and of benz(a)pyrene even 10^{-6} mg/m^3 flue gases (see Appendix Table 4 for maximum permissible PAH's-concentration in the air).

As a consequence of the air pollution and other environmental health factors an increase of cancer appeared in the last decades.

A possible reaction mechanism illustrating the cancer initiation in human organism is given in Scheme 14.1.

It is based on enzymatic processes, mostly proceeding in liver, but the oxidizing free radicals (OH, $OH_2^{\bullet-}$ etc.), generated in the organism are certainly also involved in the process. Thereby the carcinogenic PAH's-transients as well as the free radicals attack prefere ntially the unprotonated amono groups ($-NH_2$) of DNA starting the cell mutation.

On the other hand the implementation of various chlorine-containing pesticides and other chemicals as well as fertilizers in the modern agricultures, strongly contributes to the contamination of ground water /2-4/. New methods have been developed for the degradation of water pollutants. Very efficient degradation effect has been achieved by irradiation treatment (high energy electrons, γ-ray), for the decomposition of pollutants, where the combination of radiation and ozone proved to be the most successful method /5-7/.

It might be mentioned that as early as 1963 a broad correlation between electron donation capacity and carcinogenicity of some PAH's, heterocyclic-nitrogen compounds, aromatic amines and steroides was established /8/. It was also observed that some carcinogenic aromatic amines and derivatives have both properties, electron donor and acceptor.

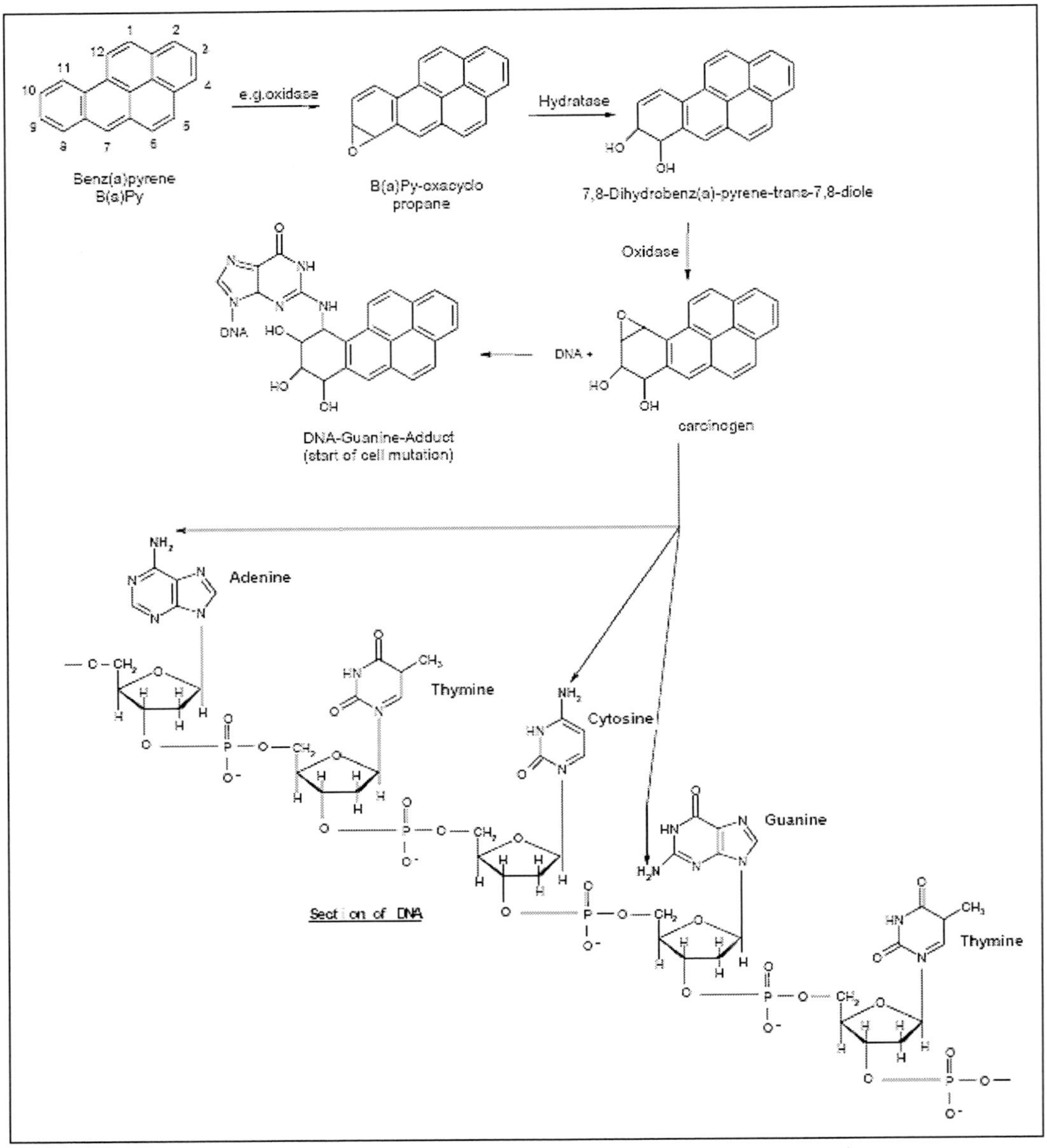

Scheme 14.1. Probable enzymatic stepwise oxidation and hydratization of benz(a)pyrene, leading to formation of DNA-guanine adduct (or/and other DNA-adducts), resulting into mutation of a cell and start of carcinogenesis.

In this respect was observed by pulse radiolysis, that pyrene can simultaneously lead to the formation of radical cations and radical anions. This unique property of pyrene may explain its extremely high carcinogenity (see Figure14.1 and Table 4 in Appendix).

In view of the present knowledge, the biological behaviour of the mentioned compounds seems to be also depending on their interaction with each other. This kind of processes are not yet clearified.

14. References

[1] Garrignes Ph. and Lamotte M.(eds.), 1991, Polycyclic Aromatic Compounds, Proceed.of the 13th Intern.Symp. on Polynuclear Aromatic Hydrocarbons, Bordeaux, France, Gordon and Breach Science, Berlin, Germany.

[2] Fishbein L.,1979, Potential Industrial Carcinogenesis and Mutagens; Elsevier, Amsterdam.

[3] Hutzinger O., Frei R.W., Merian E. and Pocchiari F.; 1982, Chlorinated Dioxines and Related Compounds – Impact on the Environment, Pergamon Press, Oxford.

[4] Strobel K. and Dieter H.J., 1990, Toxicological pick-benefit aspects of drinking water chrorination and of alternative desinfection procedures, Z.Wasser, Abwasser Forsch.23, 152-156.

[5] Getoff N., 1996, Radiation-induced degradation of water pollutants. State of the art, *Radiat.Phys.Chem.*47, 581-593.

[6] Getoff N., 2002, Factors influencing the efficiency of radiation-induced degradation of water pollutants, *Radiat.Phys.Chem.*65, 437-446.

[7] Popov P. and Getoff N., 2004, Ozonolysis and combinateion of ozonolysis and radiolysis of aqueous fluorene, *Radiat.Phys.Che.*69, 311-315.

[8] Allison A.C. and Nash T., 1963, Electron donation and acceptance by carcinogenic compounds, *Nature* 197, 758-763.

[9] Getoff N., Solar S., Richter U.-B. and Haenel M.W., 2003, Pulse radiolysis of pyrene in aprotic organic solvents. Simultanously formation of pyrene radical cations and radical anions, *Radiat.Phys.Chem.*66, 207-214.

Appendix

Table 1. Some useful physical constants and units

Avogadro constant:	$N_A = 6.0221 \times 10^{23}\ mol^{-1}$
Boltzman constant:	$k = 1.38066\ J.k^{-1}$
Faraday constant:	$F= 96.485\ C.mol^{-1}$
Gas constant:	$R = 8.3145\ J.k^{-1}$
Planck constant:	$h = 6.6261 \times 10^{-34}\ J.s$
Gray (absorbed radiation dose):	$1\ Gy = 100\ rad = 1\ J.kg^{-1}$
	$= 6.2415 \times 10^{15}\ eV.g^{-1}$
	$= 1\ W.s.kg^{-1} = 10^{-3}\ W.s.g^{-1}$
Rad (radiation absorbed dose)	$1\ rad = 100\ erg.g^{-1} = 6.24 \times 10^{13}\ eV.g^{-1}$
1 Mega-rad:	$1\ Mrad = 10^{6}\ rad = 10^{3}\ krad$
1 r (Röntgen): absorbed in air:	$1\ r = 0.873\ rad$
absorbed in water:	$1\ r = 0.970\ rad$
Joule:	$1\ J = 1\ kGy$
	$= 1\ W.s$
	$= 1 \times 10^{-7}\ erg$
Electronvolt:	$1\ eV = 1.602 \times 10^{-19}\ J$
	$1\ eV.g^{-1} = 1.602 \times 10^{-16}\ J.kg$
	$= 1.602 \times 10^{-16}\ Gy$
	$= 1.602 \times 10^{-14}\ rad$
Mega-electronenvolt:	$1\ MeV = 10^{6}\ eV = 10^{3}\ keV$
Calorie:	$1\ cal = 4.22\ J = 4.186 \times 10^{7}\ erg$
Kilocalorie per mol:	$1\ kcal.mol^{-1} = 4.3365 \times 10^{-2}\ eV.molecule^{-1}$
Kilowatt-hour:	$1\ kW.h = 8.604 \times 10^{5}\ cal_{th} = 3.60 \times 10^{6}\ J$
	$= 2.247 \times 10^{25}\ eV$
	$= 3.60 \times 10^{6}\ kg.Gy$

$1\ kWh = 1\ mA \times 1\ MeV = 3.6 \times 10^{6}\ J.kg = 360\ Mrad.kg.h^{-1}$

Table 2. Comparison the dose rate (D_R in $MGy.h^{-1}$) of various radiation sources.

Kind of Radiation Source	kW	Dose rate ($MGy.h^{-1}$)
X-rays: 10 mA, 250kV	0.5×10^{-8}	1.8×10^{-5}
^{60}Co-γ-Source		
0.5×10^{6} Curie	0.18	0.65
1.0×10^{6} Curie	0.36	1.30
Electron Accelerators:		
- Van de Graff (1 mA, 2 MeV)	2	7.2×10^{3}
- Rhodotron (20 mA, 5 MeV)	100	3.6×10^{5}
(10 mA, 10 MeV)	100	3.6×10^{5}
- DYNAMITRON (40 mA, 5 MeV)	200	7.2×10^{5}
- LINAC (50 mA, 10 MeV)	500	1.8×10^{6}
Output power of electron accelerator (in kW): 1 kW = 1 mA x 1 MeV mA = electron current; MeV = electron energy		

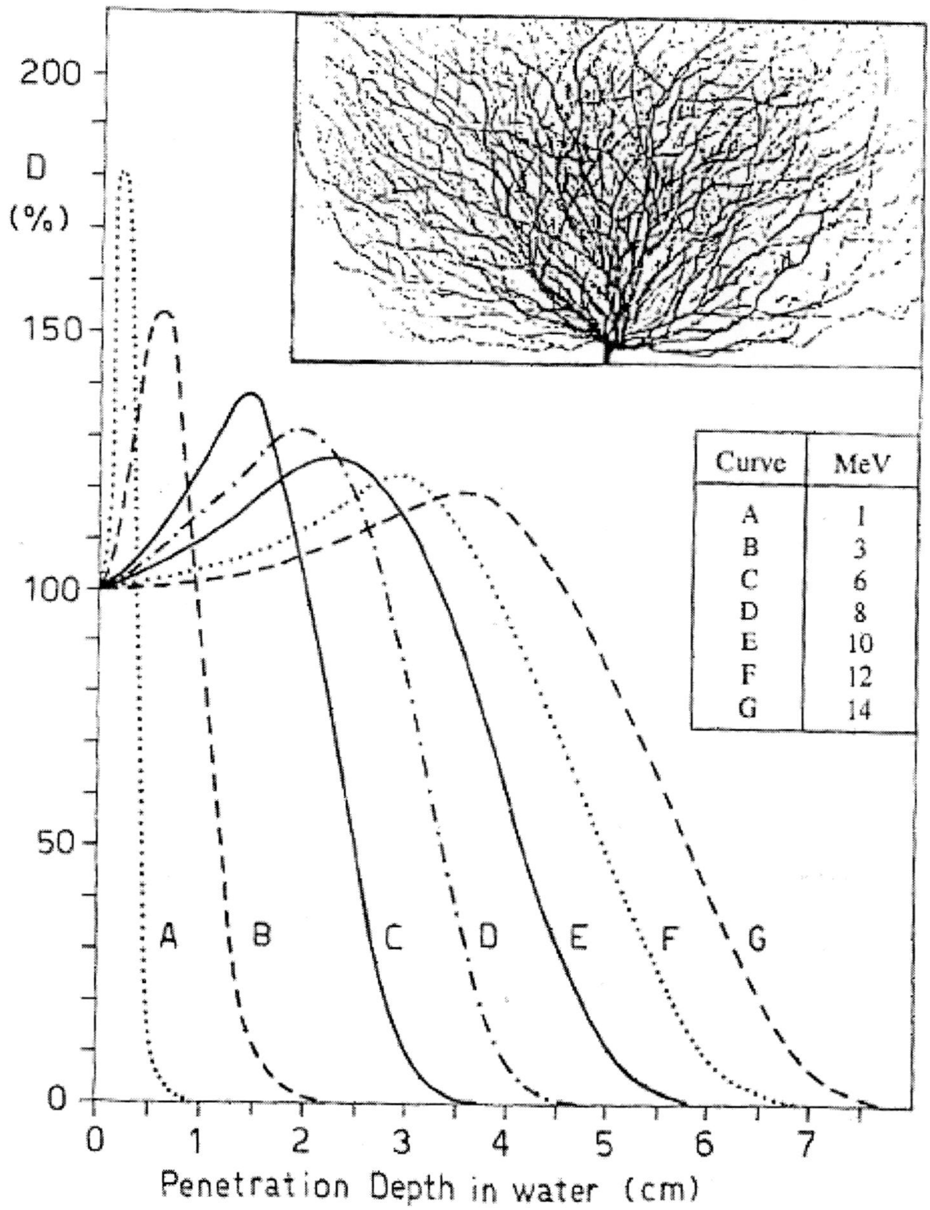

Figure 1. Depth-dose (%) distribution curves of electrons with different energies in water (valid also ≅ for tissue). Insert: Discharge traces of 3 MeV electrons (1μs pulse) in polymethyl-metacrylate.

(Reprinted from Radiat.Phys.Chem.**47**, 581-593, 1996, by N.Getoff, Radiation-induced degradation of water pollutants. State of the art, with permission from Elsevier)

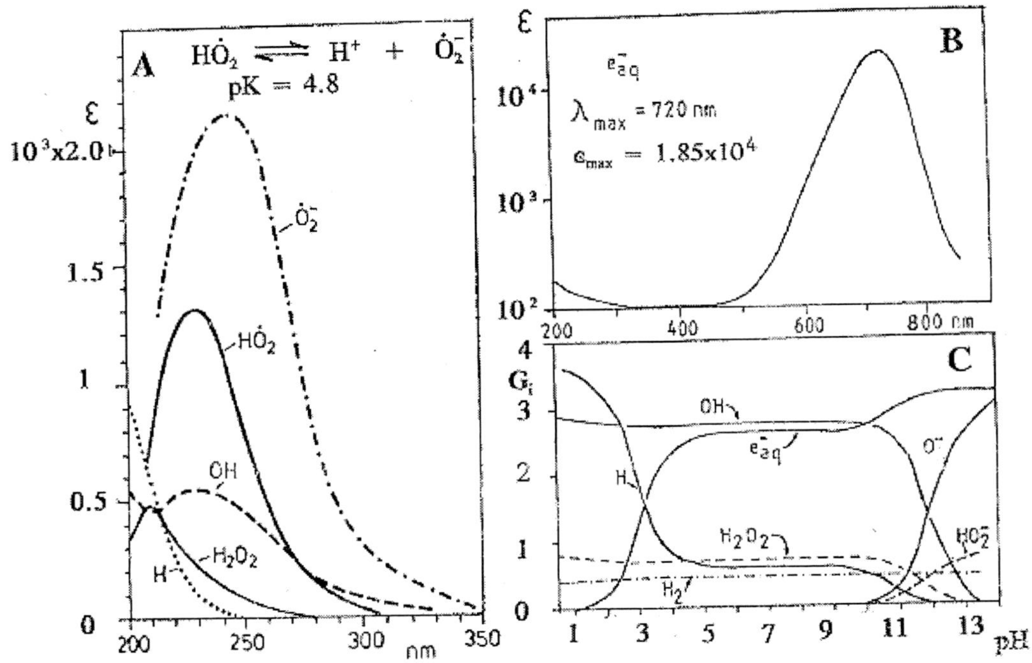

Figure 2. (A) Absorption spectra of H, OH, $HO_2^{\bullet}$ and $O_2^{\bullet-}$ radicals as well as H_2O_2 (ε in $dm^3mol^{-1}cm^{-1}$); Insert: pK-value of $HO_2^{\bullet}$.(B) Absorption spectrum of e_{aq}^- (ε in dm3mol^{-1}cm^{-1}).(C) Gi -values of the primary products of water radiolysis as a function of pH.

(Reprinted from Radiat.Phys.Chem.74, 581-593, 1996, by N.Getoff, Radiation-induced degradation of water pollutants. State of the art; with permission from Elsevier).

Table 3. Reactions and rate constants (k) of the primary products in the radiolysis of pure water

Reactions in the radiolysis of pure water	k [$dm^3.mol^{-1}.s^{-1}$]
$e^-_{aq} + H_2O \longrightarrow H + OH^-$	1.9×10^{1}
$e^-_{aq} + e^-_{aq} \longrightarrow H_2 + 2\,OH^-$	$2k = 1.1 \times 10^{10}$
$e^-_{aq} + H \longrightarrow H_2 + OH^-$	2.5×10^{10}
$e^-_{aq} + OH \longrightarrow OH^-$	3.0×10^{10}
$e^-_{aq} + O^{\bullet-} \longrightarrow 2\,OH^-$	2.2×10^{10}
$e^-_{aq} + H^+ \longrightarrow H$	2.3×10^{10}
$e^-_{aq} + H_2O_2 \longrightarrow OH^- + OH$	1.1×10^{10}
$e^-_{aq} + HO_2^- \longrightarrow 2\,OH^- + OH$	3.5×10^{9}
$e^-_{aq} + O_2 \longrightarrow O_2^{\bullet-}$	1.9×10^{10}
$e^-_{aq} + O_2^{\bullet-} \longrightarrow O_2^{2-}$	1.3×10^{10}
$H + H_2O \longrightarrow H_2 + OH$	1.0×10^{1}
$H + H \longrightarrow H_2$	$2k = 1.55 \times 10^{10}$
$H + OH \longrightarrow H_2O$	7.0×10^{9}
$H + OH^- \longrightarrow e^-_{aq}$	2.2×10^{7}
$H + H_2O_2 \longrightarrow OH + H_2O$	9.0×10^{7}
$H + O_2 \longrightarrow HO_2^{\bullet}$	2.1×10^{10}
$H + HO_2^{\bullet} \longrightarrow H_2O_2$	$\sim 10^{10}$
$OH + OH \longrightarrow H_2O_2$	$2k = 1.1 \times 10^{10}$
$OH + O^{\bullet-} \longrightarrow HO_2^-$	$\sim 2 \times 10^{10}$
$OH + H_2 \longrightarrow H + H_2O$	4.2×10^{7}
$OH + OH^- \longrightarrow O^{\bullet-} + H_2O$	1.3×10^{10}
$OH + H_2O_2 \longrightarrow H_2O + HO_2^{\bullet}$	2.7×10^{7}
$OH + HO_2^{\bullet-} \longrightarrow OH^- + HO_2^{\bullet}$	7.5×10^{9}
$OH + H_2O_2^+ \longrightarrow H_3O^+ + O_2$	1.2×10^{10}
$OH + HO_2^{\bullet} \longrightarrow H_2O + O_2$	6×10^{9}
$OH + O_2^{\bullet-} \longrightarrow OH^- + O_2$	8×10^{9}
$O^{\bullet-} + H_2O \longrightarrow OH^- + OH$	1.8×10^{6}
$O^{\bullet-} + O^{\bullet-} \longrightarrow O_2^{2-}$	
$O^{\bullet-} + H_2 \longrightarrow H + OH$	8.0×10^{7}
$O^{\bullet-} + H_2O_2 \longrightarrow O_2^{\bullet-} + H_2O$	5×10^{8}
$O^{\bullet-} + HO_2^- \longrightarrow O_2^{\bullet-} + OH^-$	4×10^{8}
$O^{\bullet-} + O_2 \longrightarrow O_3^-$	3.6×10^{9}
$O^{\bullet-} + O_2 \longrightarrow 2\,OH^- + O_2$	6.0×10^{8}

(Reprinted from: "Critical Review of Rate Constants for Reaction of Hydrated Electrons, Hydrogen Atoms and Hydroxyl Radicals in Aqueous Solution" by G.V.Buxton, C.L.Greenstock, W.P. Helman and A.B:Ross, J.Phys.Chem.Ref.Data **17**, 513-886, 1988; with permission from Publisher).

Table 4. Maximum permissible concentration of some polycyclic aromatic hydrocarbons (PAHs) formed by combustion of fossils fuels

Name	Formula	Max. permissible concentration (mg/m^3 flue gas)
Acenaphtene	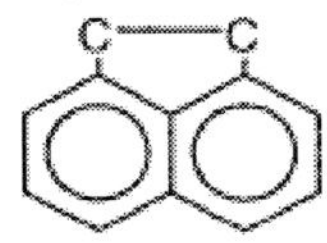	0,07
Naphtalene	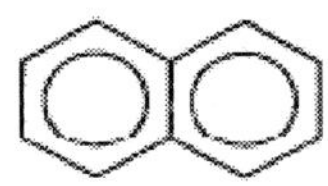	0,052
Fluorene	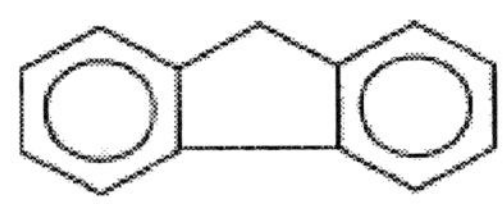	0,002
Diphenyloxide (Diphenylether)	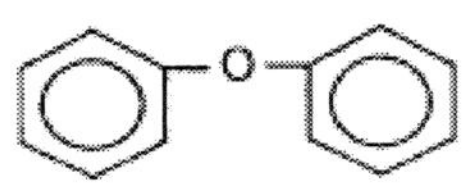	0,03
Anthracene	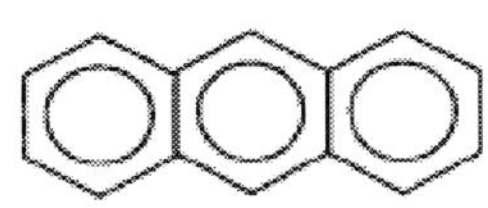	0,001
Fluoranthene	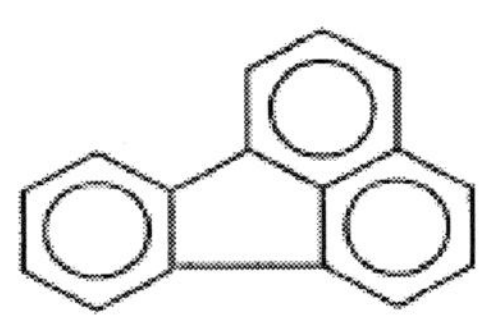	0,001
Pyrene	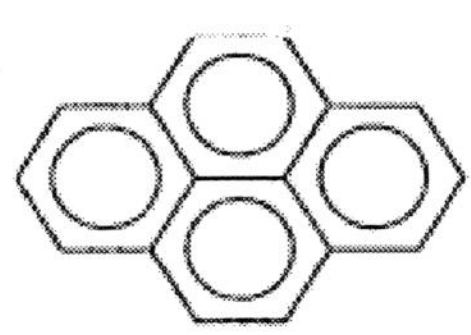	0,001
Benzo(A)pyrene	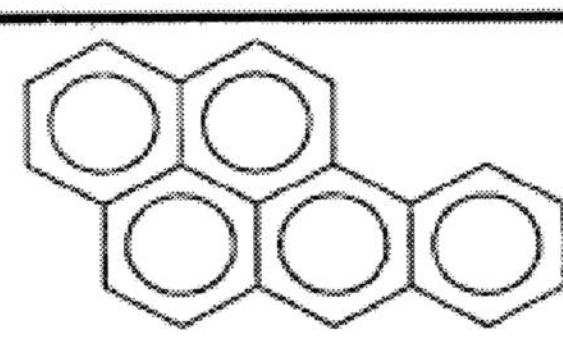	0,000001

Table 5. Recommended books

1. **Introduction to Radiation Chemistry,** 3rd Ed.
   J.W.T.Spinks and R.J.Woods
   John Wiley & Sons Inc., USA; 1990.
2. **Fundamentals in Radiation Chemistry,**
   A.Mozumder, Academic Press, 1999
3. **Radiation Chemistry. Principals and Application,**
   I.Farhataziz, M.A.J.Rodgers (Eds.)
   VCH Publishers, Inc.; Weinheim, Germany, 1987.
4. **Flash Photolysis and Pulse Radiolysis,**
   R.V.Bensasson, E.J.Land, T,G,Truscott,
   Pergamon Press, Oxford, 1983.
5. **An Introduction to Radiobiology,** 2nd Ed.
   A.H.W.Nias; John Wiley & Sons, Inc., USA.
6. **Introduction to Radiobiology,**
   M.Tubiana, J.Dutreix, A.Wamberrie,
   Taylor and Francis, London, 1990.
7. **Biological Radiation Effects,**
   J.Kiefer; Springer Verlag, Berlin, 1990.
8. **Free Radicals in Biology and Medicine,** 3rd Ed.
   B.Halliwell, J.M.C.Cutteridge,
   Oxford University Press, 2005.
9. **Free Radical – Induced DNA-Damage and its Repair. A Chemical Perspective,**
   C.von Sonntag; Springer Verlag, Berlin, 2006

Index

B

C

D

E

F

G

K

L

M

Q

R

S

T

U

V

W

X

Y